WELL & GOOD

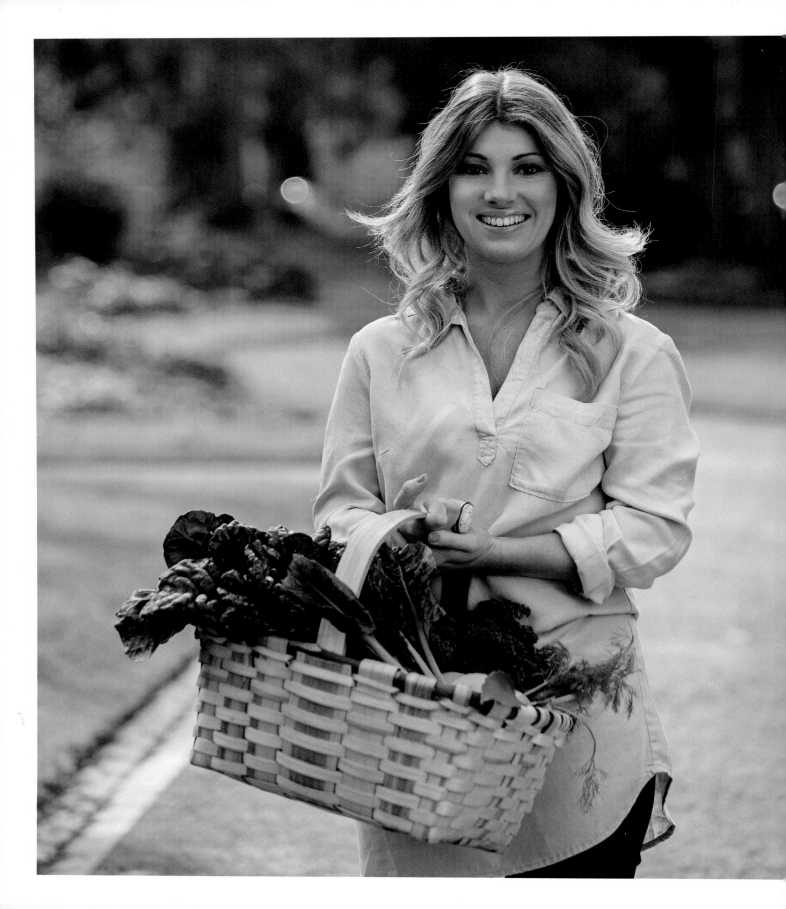

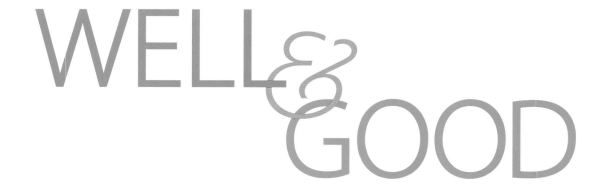

WELL & GOOD

SUPERCHARGE YOUR HEALTH
FOR FERTILITY & WELLNESS

Nat KRINGOUDIS

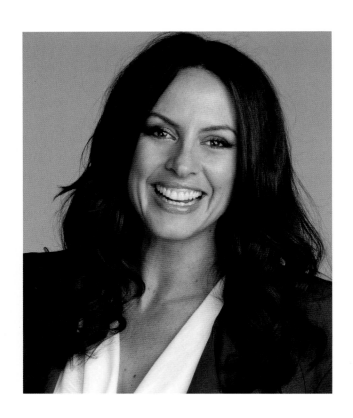

FOREWORD

As a woman in her late thirties I know all too well the importance of taking charge of your fertility. I think we grow up thinking that getting pregnant is something that will just happen. And if there are problems, medicine will fix them. But the path to pregnancy—and true wellness—is not so passive. Taking it into your own hands is also simpler and far more empowering!

Several years ago I got quite unwell with an autoimmune disease (that affected my female hormones dramatically). It was my wake-up call and in a way I'm grateful that it

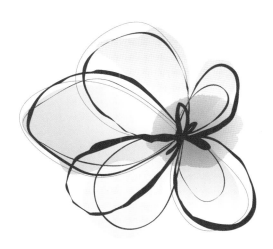

happened. It got me to take charge. Taking charge of your health is not as onerous as it sounds. In fact, I found it an enlivening and rewarding journey. It took some time, and some trialling of different techniques, until I found what worked for me, but once I did, I started to get instant results.

Taking charge of your fertility is about figuring out what works for you. For me, this involved experimenting, and through a range of techniques I got to a space where my body began to feel balanced and well. Truly well. Nutrition was key, and this is something that Nat espouses wisely and simply.

Acupuncture worked wonders. Getting my sleep patterns regulated saw results. So did a number of lifestyle choices geared at getting me gently aware and receptive to my body. I chronicle these regularly on my blog.

This is the other thing. Taking charge of your fertility is also about taking charge of your life. The principles that worked for me and that Nat outlines in this book aren't just about getting pregnant … they're about getting well and happy. There is no quick fix. It is a journey, but one that pays off. You can start the journey right now, by reading this book.

Be well,
Sarah Wilson
Journalist, TV host and wellness blogger

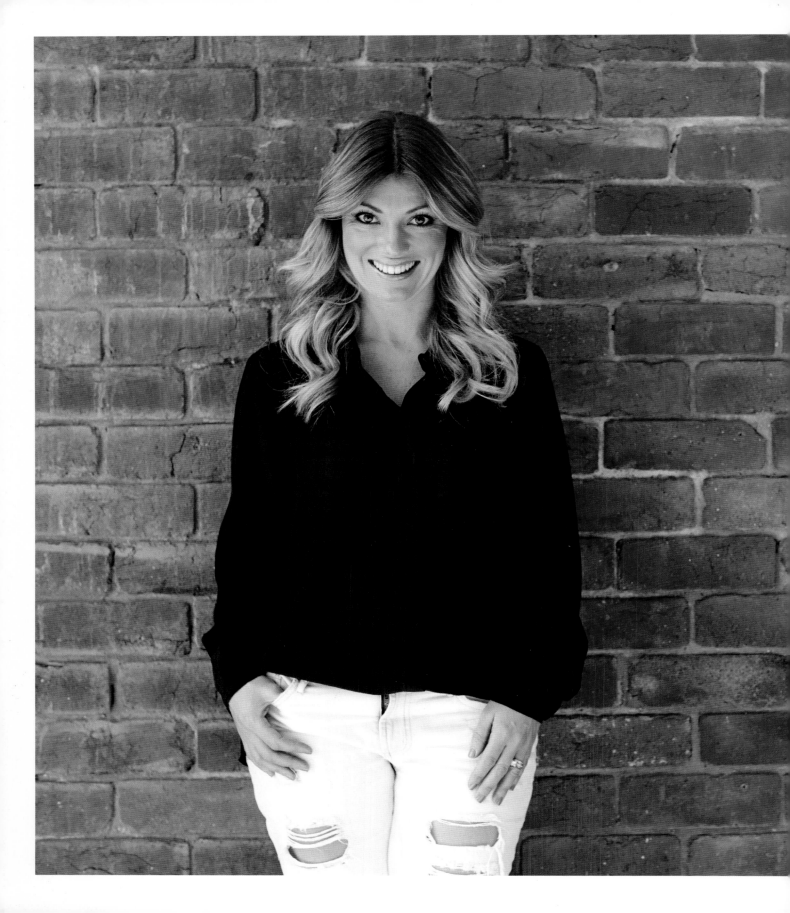

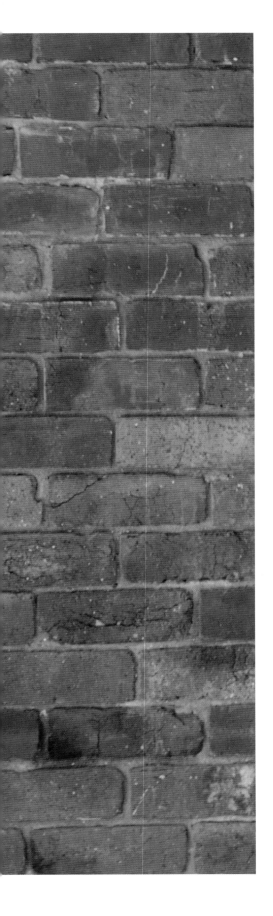

ABOUT THE AUTHOR

𝓃at Kringoudis is a Chinese medicine practitioner, acupuncturist, natural fertility educator and author. She's also the owner of The Pagoda Tree, a hub for natural fertility and women's health in Australia.

Natalie recognised the large gap between conventional medicine and wellness support and has developed a unique approach to natural fertility—integrating western medical science with alternative therapies, Chinese medicine and natural fertility methods.

Nat seeks to inspire others in their path towards wellness and to educate women on how their choices shape their reproductive health; she hopes to reach not only those embarking on parenthood but also women at different stages of life. For Nat, fertility isn't just about babies, it's about outstanding health.

Nat shares her specialist insight on her
WEBSITE www.natkringoudis.com.au
TWITTER Nat Kringoudis
FACEBOOK Nat Kringoudis
INSTAGRAM NatKringoudis

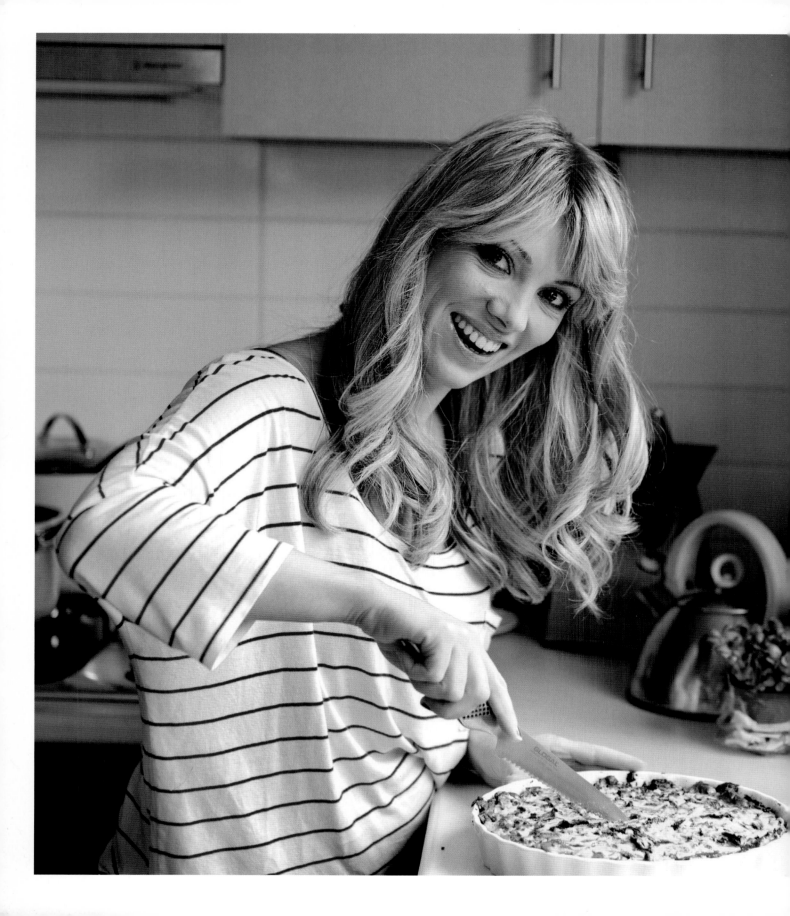

CONTENTS

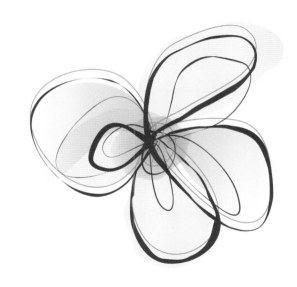

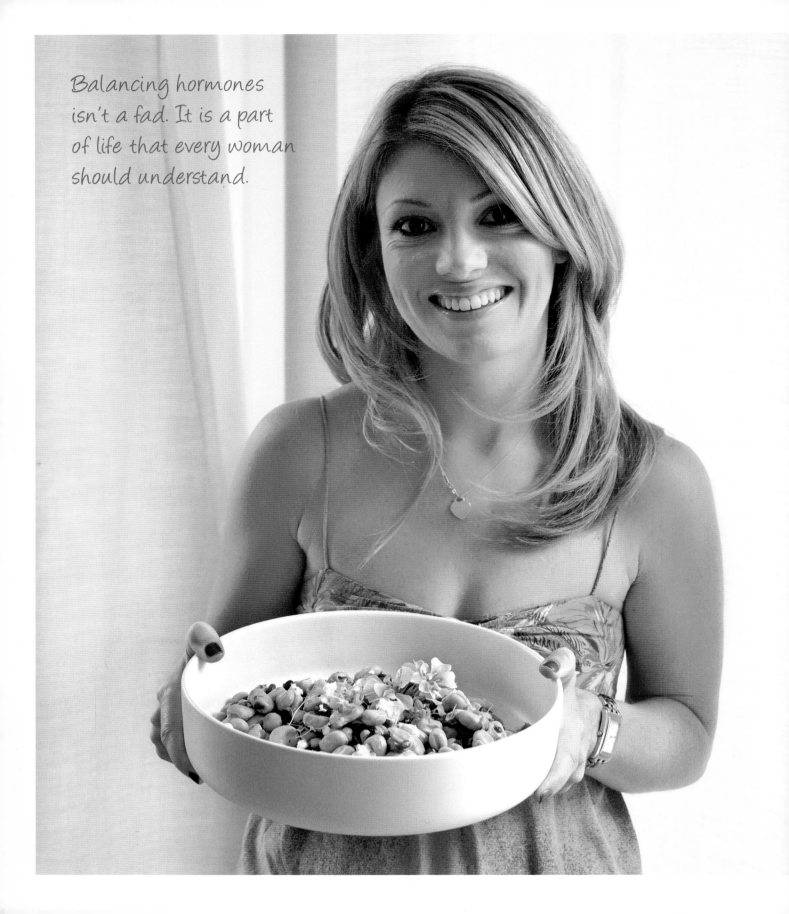

Balancing hormones isn't a fad. It is a part of life that every woman should understand.

INTRODUCTION

Before you eat, do you think about the nutritional value of your meal?
You wouldn't be alone if the answer was no.

My intention when I set out to write this book was to give women (and men) all the information they needed to prepare their bodies to go on and make amazingly healthy little people. But in the process I discovered something. Those trying for a baby don't actually need to be convinced to put their best foot forward. Sure, some women I see are in a mess health-wise and need advice—and that's my job. But where I can actually be most useful is in reaching out to the younger generation, so that they can be laying the foundations of a healthy hormonal life instead of playing catch-up later.

We have the ability to heal our bodies under almost all circumstances, and with the right knowledge we can start making informed decisions around diet and lifestyle. This is where the journey towards a fertile future starts.

When we eat, many of us think only about taste. There's nothing wrong with enjoying your food and satisfying your tastebuds. Food that is nutritious and delicious is what it's all about.

Food makes all the difference. In my clinic I regularly see patients who are fuelling their bodies on the equivalent of cardboard. How they expect it to flourish baffles me, although I'm not sure they have actually stopped and thought about what they could or should be doing to improve the situation.

Have you ever grown fruit or vegetables from a seed? It is a complex process. You need to prepare the soil, plant the seed, water it frequently, feed it, water it some more, though not too much, and if you've done the job properly, you might end up with a reward for your labour: food! But if you haven't done the necessary preparation, it's unlikely you'll produce anything.

Your body isn't any different. To create happy hormones and an all-round, well-working body, you need to provide it with the same level of care as a veggie patch. You need to do the groundwork. You need to fertilise yourself.

Today, the rate of infertility is climbing rapidly. Among the many hurdles on the road to healthy hormones these are some of the most common experienced by my clients:

- polycystic ovarian syndrome (PCOS)
- endometriosis
- missing periods (amenorrhea)
- recurrent miscarriage
- thyroid troubles
- adrenal fatigue
- weight-control issues.

I'm constantly asked to comment on why I think this is happening. There are so many factors—many we can't necessarily control—from chemicals in our food and pesticides in our water, poor air quality and other environmental factors, to the cleaning products we scrub our showers with. We must focus on what we can control: the food we eat and the lifestyle we live.

The gut is the pivot of our health—you might be excited to learn that you're going to discover how to love your gut on a whole new level. The Chinese recognised several thousand years ago how imperative excellent digestive function is and established that there is a direct relationship between our gut and our health.

Your gut:
- supports good immunity
- refreshes and cleans out your blood
- fuels your body as food is digested
- puts the good bits—vitamins and minerals—back into the body
- sends out the unwanted matter as waste.

When this pivotal system is out of balance, we see toxic build-up in parts of the body where it isn't meant to be. Toxins bank up our digestive systems like a blocked sewerage pipe, making it sluggish and fighting to work properly.

When we are run down, the body flicks the off switch on the systems it doesn't need to survive. This is a survival mechanism. And the first to be popped off the perch is the reproductive system; it just isn't a vital function. When the body is in such a state of disarray there is no way it can reproduce, nor would it be very desirable. An unhealthy body will not make healthy babies. An unhealthy body calls for mission overhaul! But before we go on, it's important to remember: fertility isn't just about babies, even if that's the point we're working towards. Fertility is about a thriving reproductive system, free from hormone imbalance, menstrual issues, conditions such as PCOS, endometriosis, thyroid issues and a whole swag of other symptoms. It is about a thriving body.

To help you achieve this goal, I will share with you some of my favourite hormone-boosting recipes and also assist you to come to a whole new way of understanding and fuelling your body. I have the knowledge and you have the power: together we make a great team!

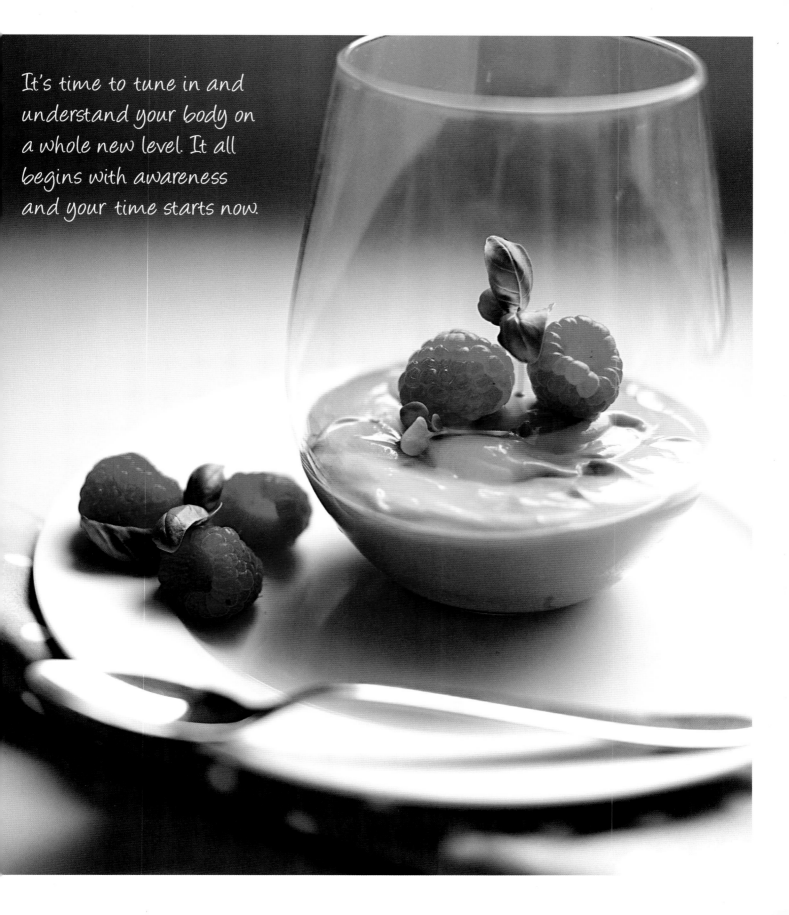

It's time to tune in and understand your body on a whole new level. It all begins with awareness and your time starts now.

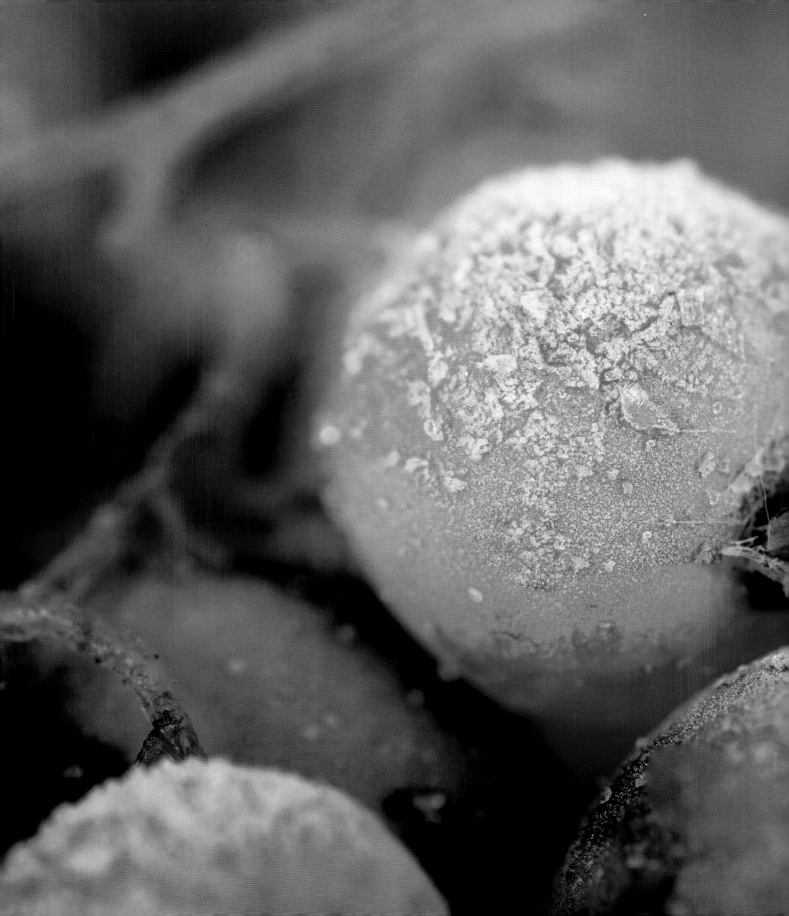

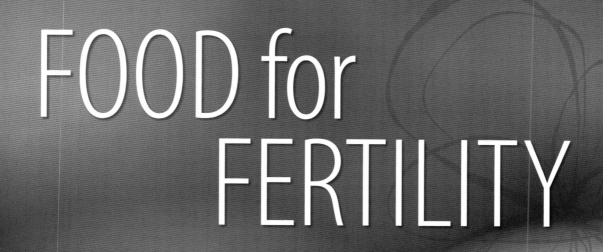

FOOD for
FERTILITY

FOOD for FERTILITY

I suspect that our forebears had a whole lot more intuitive knowledge about nutrition than we give them credit for. Sure, they didn't have labs to nut out exactly what foods contained, but they had a sound knowledge of the medicinal uses of food. They ate to fuel the body, to nourish and to heal.

They realised, by observation, that some foods worked really well together and others were fizzers. They listened to their bodies and figured out how to eat and even came up with theories on why. How? Well, they had the time. Time to stop and observe. On top of that—food didn't come wrapped in plastic. It was eaten exactly as intended—whole. No skim milk (seriously!) or low-fat mayonnaise, and they weren't fat either! They ate to live, and as a result they were a whole lot more fertile than we are today.

Pump up the fat! It's not fat that makes you 'fat'. Okay, so don't start hoeing down chunks of lard (although even lard can be okay if you eat it in the right way), but what you'll come to understand is that refined foods, packaged foods, sugars and saturated fats are what is making us sick, tired and ... fat!

Let's Break It Down

Consider this a rough dietary guide to maintaining healthy reproductive function:

50% protein (animal or vegetable)

20% quality, low-GI carbohydrates

30% healthy fats

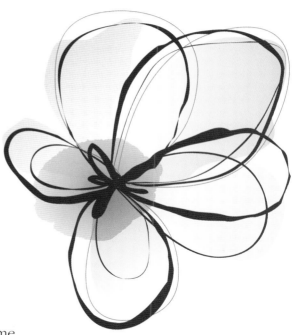

Eating for fertility isn't rocket science. All it involves is some common sense and understanding. At my clinic, The Pagoda Tree, we don't apply a one-size-fits-all approach to treatment, but we do encourage certain ways of eating that will benefit your hormonal health. These principles are the same for everyone—we were all designed to eat for health.

I encourage you to start unlearning the diet thinking that has become the norm since the 1980s. In fact, put it away with your hypercolour t-shirts and your legwarmers. It doesn't work and it sets you up for failure. Proteins and fats are the most important foods for fertility and health, because our hormones are made from them.

Fat doesn't equal fat. Sugar, on the other hand, chucks on the weight faster than you can finish your lollipop or pop another scoop into your coffee. To boost your fertility you need to be substituting sugar with protein and fat.

We need to make some changes—that means cutting down on all refined sugars and carbohydrates—and ramping up the intake of healthy fats and quality proteins. Your body converts high-GI carbohydrates to sugar and then stores it as fat to

Healthy fats go gangbusters on your well being and fertility. These include omega-3 and omega-6 (found in fish and eggs), polyunsaturated fats, found in seeds and nuts, and saturated fats, found in meats and coconut products.

Quality protein such as that found in foods like salmon or eggs is the key. Grabbing the nearest jar of protein powder will not cut the mustard.

protect itself from the potential damage caused by these dangerously high levels of sugar. This is toxic and bad news for health and fertility. You might think to yourself—how can so many sugary and high-GI foods be accepted in our western diets if they are so toxic? Through genetic modification and processing, our foods are not what they were fifty years ago.

Natural foods are not meant to be played around with. Messing around has consequences—and here we are, suffering majorly. We thought we could outsmart nature by manipulating food to yield greater profit. We are now paying the price for modified foods—the state of our health reflects the blunder we've made.

Skim and low-fat varieties of milk are the worst kind. Remember, whole foods are what nature intended us to eat. When we cut the fat from milk what's left is the sugar content. This also makes it more difficult to digest. My advice? Don't touch it.

Protein for Youthfulness

A diet high in refined carbohydrates (high GI) and low in fats and proteins leads to premature aging. This type of diet often comes with the calorie-counting approach to weight control. Low protein intake leads to the breaking down of muscle tissue—a significant marker of aging.

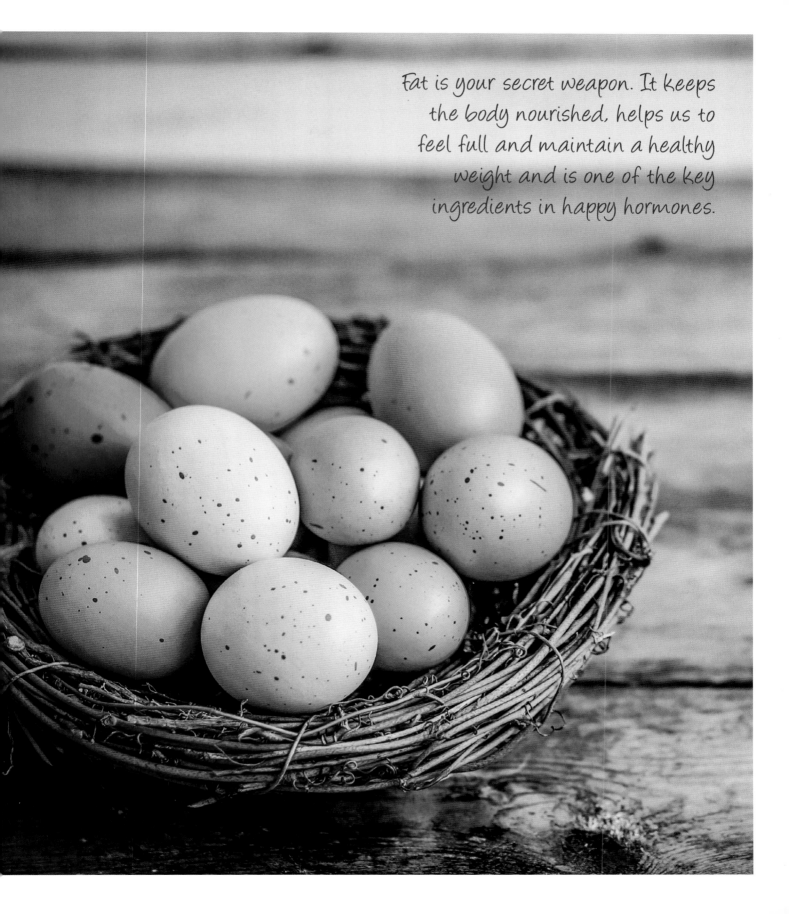

Fat is your secret weapon. It keeps the body nourished, helps us to feel full and maintain a healthy weight and is one of the key ingredients in happy hormones.

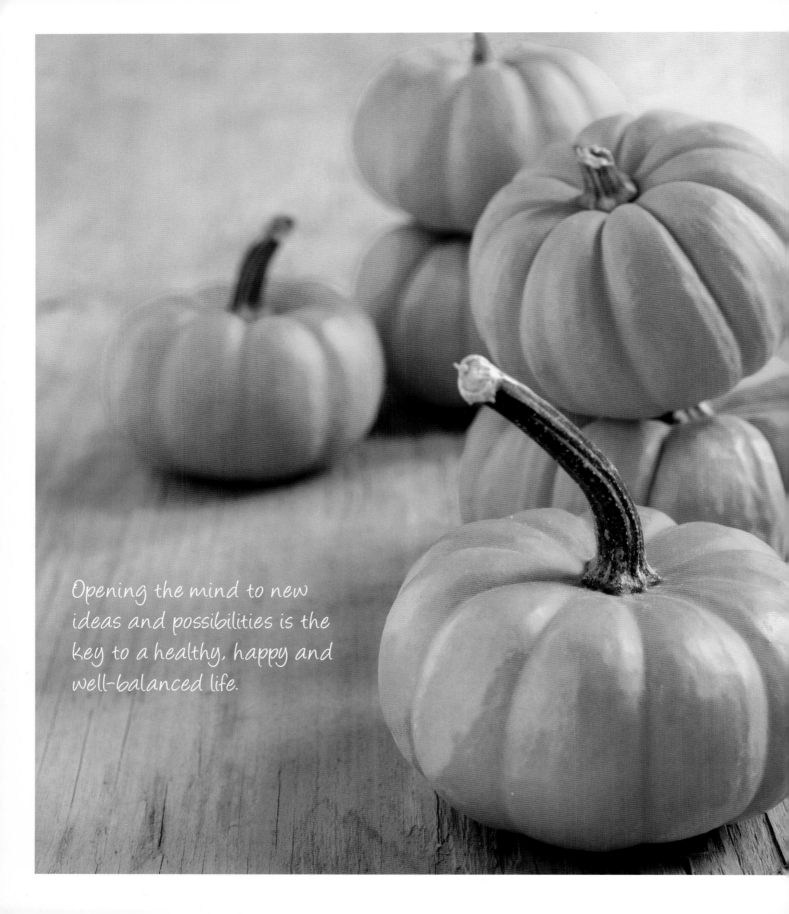

Opening the mind to new ideas and possibilities is the key to a healthy, happy and well-balanced life.

Those with gluten intolerance or coeliac disease need to pay particular attention to the foods they eat, as the gut health is reflected in fertility. Gluten will inflame most guts—making digestion sluggish and impairing absorption of vital nutrients. Found in wheat, rye and barley, gluten sets off a reaction causing damage to the lining of the gut, effectively leaving it unable to absorb the nutrients from food.

No nutrients, no fuel, no fertility.

Gluten intolerance and coeliac disease can be the cause for recurrent conception problems. Given the high cost of testing for these conditions, I advise simply trying a new way of eating for a few months to allow you to realise how much better you can feel when avoiding gluten (and why not cut out sugar for good measure?!).

The good news is, when you eat for fertility, you are actually eating the perfect gluten-free or coeliac diet. Everybody benefits from this way of eating. We will learn much more about the gut as we go. You'll quickly discover that the key to health is loving your gut!

When you eliminate gluten you will notice positive changes, including weight loss, more energy, a sense of 'lightness', less bloating, consistent bowel movements and emotional balance.

Your fertility is an extension of your health.

Interestingly, from the perspective of Chinese medicine, the heart and the uterus have a very strong relationship. What does this mean for us in the west? Simple. Your emotions will affect your fertility. This is important for couples who have been trying to conceive for some time, and especially relevant to couples using in vitro fertilisation (IVF). Over time, IVF may begin to affect how a woman feels, resulting in poor quality eggs and less response to fertility drugs.

IVF places massive strain on the body and the emotions—your emotional health will considerably affect your success in IVF.

When the body recognises harmful substances (i.e. refined foods, high-GI carbohydrates and gluten) it goes into a fat-storing frenzy, producing adipose tissue (aka fat) to trap the toxins and tuck them out of harm's way. Eat the wrong foods every day and this toxic fat builds up. Your gut becomes impaired and it can't get on with its work, leaving you nutritionally depleted, not to mention with a few extra kilos.

Chinese medicine recognises just how depleting IVF can be, as it drains the body of vital blood and nutrients. The Chinese understand that the heart propels the blood through the ren channel (the midline of the body) to nourish the uterus and ensure a healthy menstrual cycle, including the quality of eggs. With depleted blood, the health of the reproductive system suffers. But the impact isn't limited to the physical—the organs are also emotional centres in the body. Given this connection between the heart and the uterus, it is vital that IVF patients have emotional support. In my experience this yields amazing results.

Acupuncture and Chinese medicine are also known to increase the success of assisted conception. Eating for fertility will also be vital for these couples, to nourish the reproductive system and the entire body.

Now that we have established that to eat yourself to fertility you need to increase protein and fat and decrease sugar and gluten, you know the secret to experiencing wellness like never before.

If the idea of limiting your gluten and sugar feels overwhelming, try focusing on what you can have rather than on what you can't. With this positive outlook and some wonderful recipes you will feel so great you won't miss them at all!

TOP TEN
FERTILE FOODS

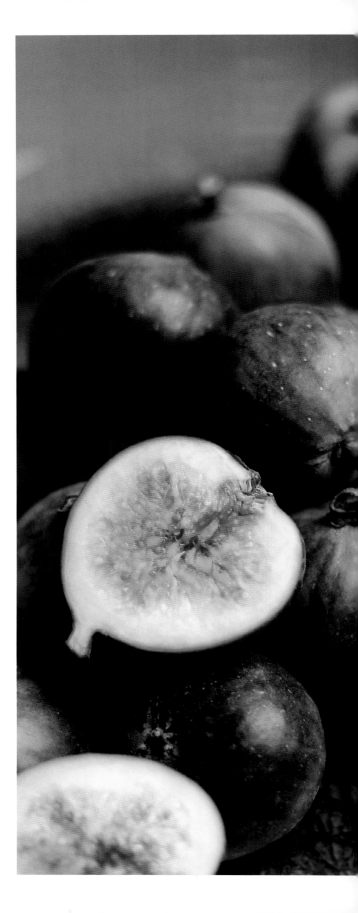

❶ EGGS
the ace of spades when it comes to fertility, they are the complete meal (protein plus good-quality fats), beautifully packaged in their own little shell.

❷ AVOCADO
balances hormones and benefits female reproductive organs. A wonderful source of therapeutic fats.

❸ FIGS
great for treating the male reproductive system and boosting semen quality.

❹ GREEN TEA
cleanses and increases fertility by benefitting fertile mucus.

❺ MACA
this superfood should be your best friend. It balances hormones and eases symptoms of pre-menstrual syndrome (PMS).

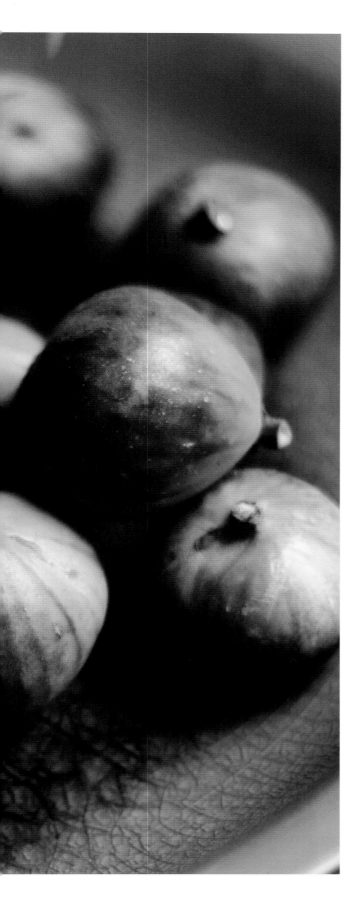

⑥ BEANS

high in protein and essential vitamins
and minerals, including zinc, iron and biotin.

⑦ NUTS

go nuts with nuts. They measure high on
the protein and therapeutic fats gauge.
But they must be soaked (see Recipes).

⑧ WILD SALMON

full of omega-3, fatty acids, high-quality protein,
B12 and iron: all essential for overall health.

⑨ COCONUT CREAM

high in quality fats and electrolytes—coconut
cream gets your tummy working. High in
antimicrobial properties, it's like having
a chimney sweeper for your insides!

⑩ OLIVES

cells are changed by stress, but the antioxidants
in olives can help repair the damage, assisting
you in maintaining a healthy reproductive system.

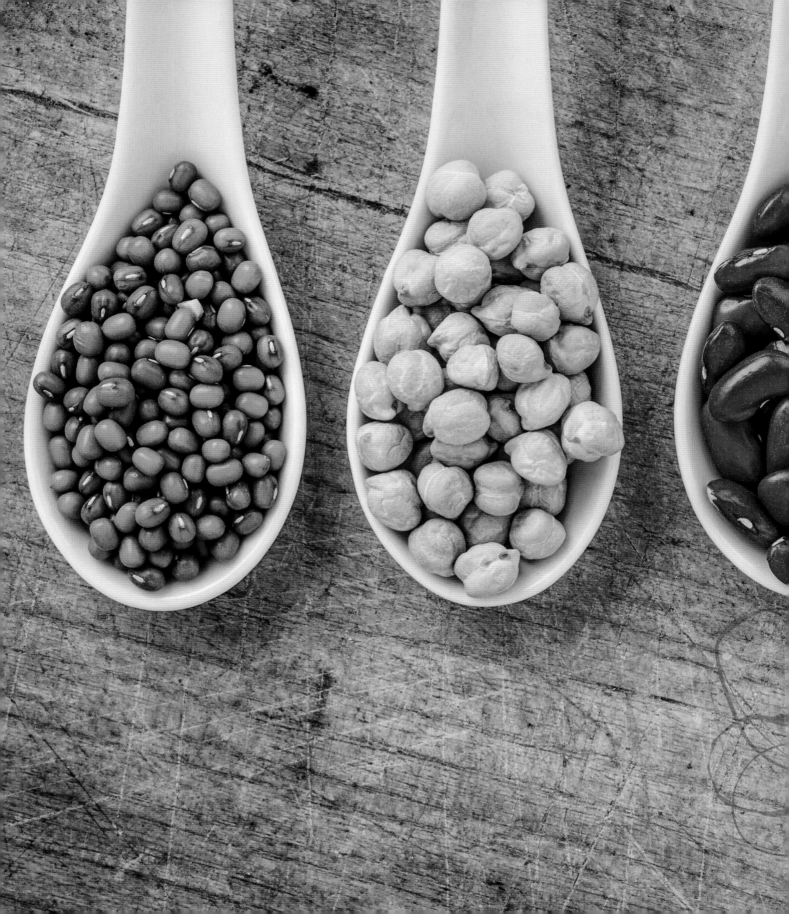

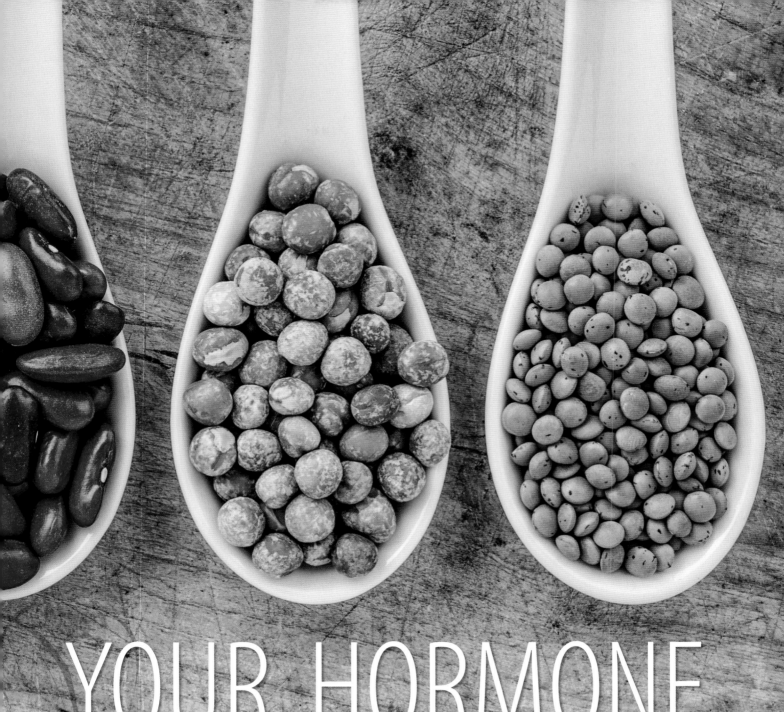

YOUR HORMONE HAPPY BODY

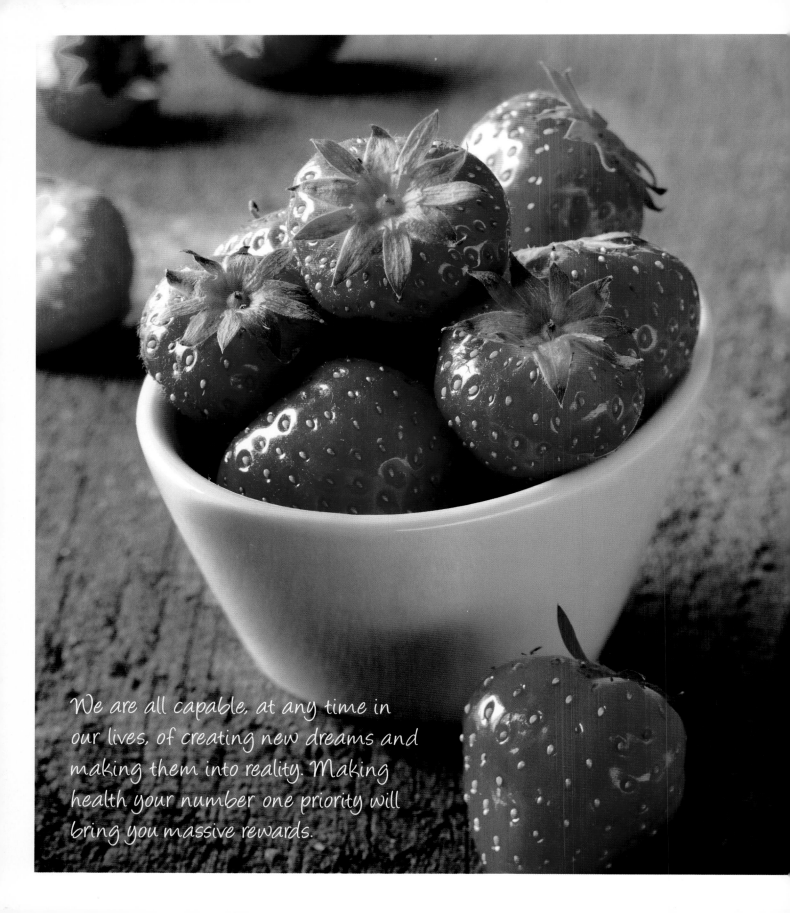

We are all capable, at any time in our lives, of creating new dreams and making them into reality. Making health your number one priority will bring you massive rewards.

YOUR HORMONE HAPPY BODY

As we have seen there are certain conditions and illnesses that can stand between you and your more fertile self—endometriosis, PCOS, hormone imbalances, thyroid issues and coeliac disease are the main culprits. Unfortunately, the absence of these illnesses doesn't mean you're in the clear—if it's wellness you want, you'll have to make some changes.

Everyone will benefit from the fertility diet—and while it may not completely resolve a specific condition, it will undoubtedly improve health—in many cases so much so that conception is no longer a problem.

Those of you experiencing fertility complications will now be starting to see why it's so important to fuel your body well—remember the seed metaphor—and maybe you have also started to realise how if the soil (your body) is incredibly nutrient rich this will flow into the health of your growing child.

Beyond nutrition and diet, there are some very important factors we need to look at. What follows are ten key areas that need to be addressed for happy hormones.

Ten Steps to Wellness

❶ Weight

Weight is a major contributor to fertility. To maintain a normal reproductive cycle, it is important that you have a healthy proportion of body fat. If you are overweight or underweight please don't roll your eyes or throw the book across the room. Eating for fertility will help you get your weight to exactly where it should be, for you.

A decrease in body fat in a lean person (as little as 10%) can be enough to delay menstruation or inhibit ovulation, and that's bad news for fertility. Your menstrual cycle relies on a certain regularity: approximately a twenty-eight-day cycle. Your follicular phase (from the start of menstruation to ovulation) needs to be a minimum of eleven days to ensure the egg is fully grown and released at the appropriate time. The same goes for your luteal phase (from ovulation to menstruation). To achieve the right hormonal environment, this should also be no less than eleven days. If your menstrual cycle runs short, you may very well be inhibiting your fertility. If it runs long it's less problematic, but it's still important to establish why. Over the year, long menstrual cycles also equate to fewer chances to conceive! We will dig into effortless weight adjustment and better understanding of ovulation in later chapters, but right now it's important just to understand that weight plays an integral role in hormone health and fertility.

In underweight females, the secretion of gondadotropin-releasing hormone (GnRH) by the hypothalamus is abnormal in quantity and timing, leading to low levels of the hormones that stimulate the ovaries to make and release the egg (follicle-stimulating hormone and luteinising hormone). Thus, because of low oestrogen and progesterone, the follicles (or eggs) on the ovaries fail to develop properly. It's a hormonal nightmare! Women with this condition may have their period as frequently as every fourteen days, and unfortunately this often isn't long enough for a fertile cycle.

Exactly the same goes for overweight women. Hormones are frequently out of balance, which affects fertility. Weight loss of as little as 4 kilograms can be enough to get back to fertility.

Men—don't think you're off the hook! Your weight will also affect the motility and density (quality) of your sperm and, of course, your health on the whole.

For this reason it is vital that you—women and men—gear towards your 'fertile weight'.

Creating a healthier, optimal body isn't about being skinny; it's about being in a place of optimal wellness—thriving as a nourished woman.

Fertile Weight Calculator

Your body mass index (BMI) can be confusing and sometimes the figures are way out. There's an easy way to determine your optimal fertile weight—subtract 100 from your height. So if you are 156 centimetres (like me) your ideal fertile weight is around 56 kilograms. Remember, this is just a guide to move you toward your more fertile weight and will vary slightly from person to person.

Obese and underweight women are at risk of miscarriage, gestational diabetes and hypertension, premature delivery, stillbirth and low birth weight. So you can see how important your weight can be—it will set you up for a healthy pregnancy and also ensure that you don't have too many kilograms to lose post birth.

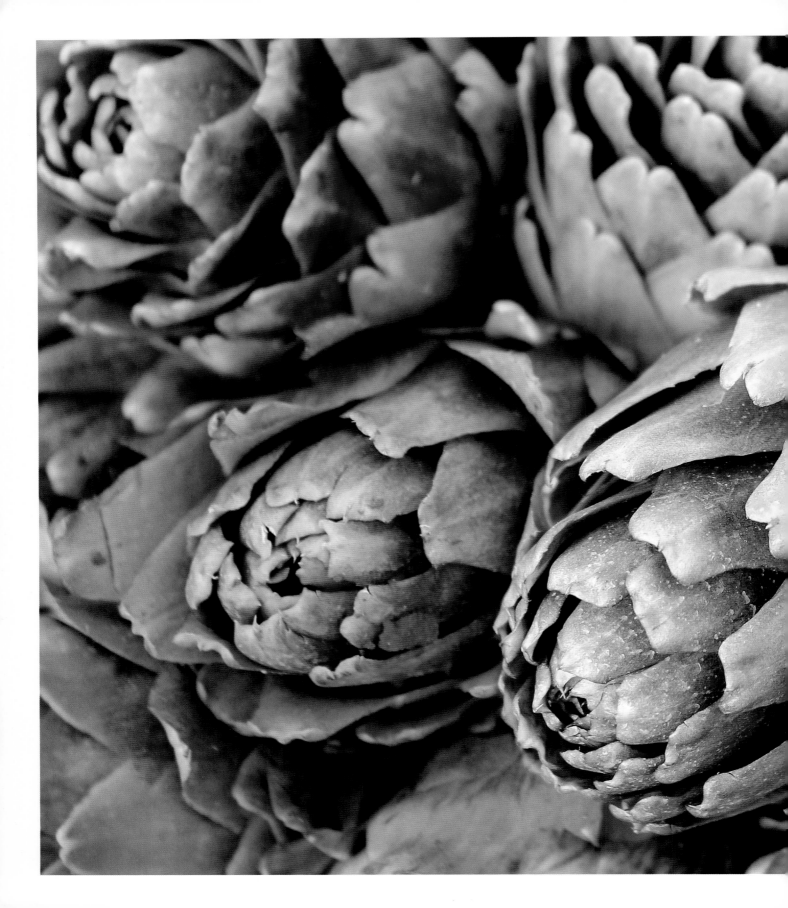

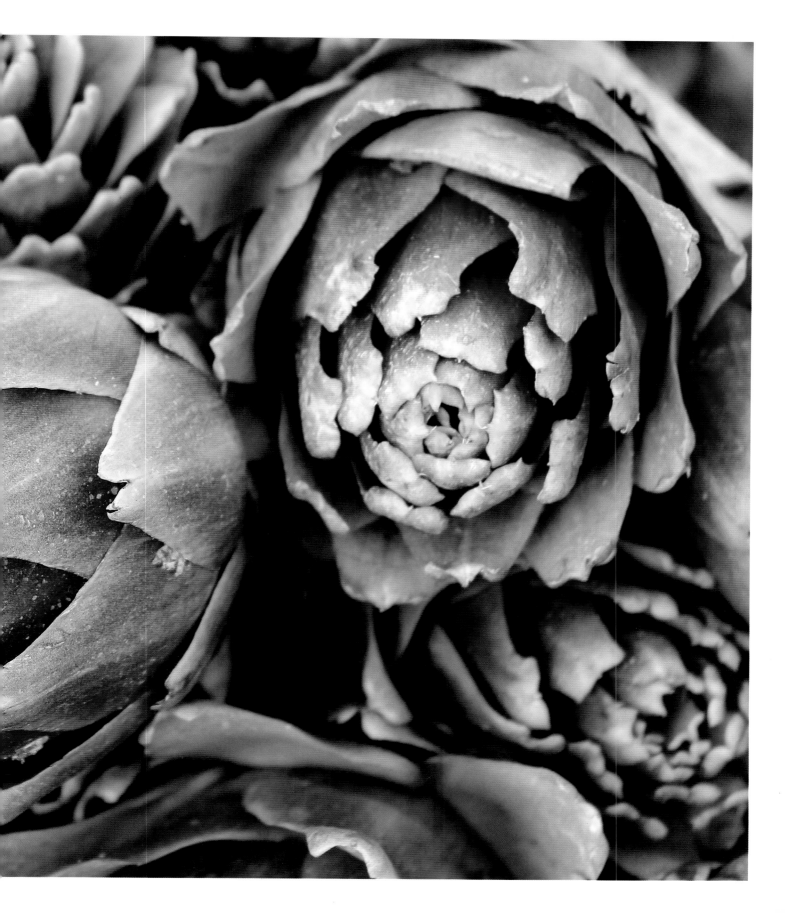

❷ Sleep

Stress and lack of rest (specifically sleep) upsets every part of our inner workings. We know how awful and exhausted we feel when we are stressing more and resting less. Go long enough without adequate rest and you will notice how your skin dries out and your eyes sink.

It's fair to say that what's happening on the outside is likely to be mirrored in the reproductive system. It will literally be dry and sunken and heading towards barren. Not only will you feel lousy if you are sleep deprived, but your body will not be functioning as it should. When we fail to listen to the warning bells, we can't expect great health.

Think of your eight hours rest as time-travelling to breakfast!

Sleep between the hours of 10pm and 6am. This will help get hormone levels to where they should be.

Our bodies run on a 24-hour cycle known as the circadian rhythm. This is the body's inner timekeeper, responsible for the day-to-day (and night) bodily functions. One of its main jobs is regulating hormone production. The eyes are receptive to light changes, which are detected in the brain, sending messages to the circadian clock. When light decreases, our clock tells us it is time to rest, and when light increases we start to awaken.

Regular disruption to these patterns will most certainly affect your body's normal working order—fertility included. This is particularly relevant for shift workers, as their inner timekeeper is generally compromised. Hormone secretion is controlled to a large degree by the circadian clock, and sleep is one of the major things that will affect this—we need to sleep at the right time.

Here's some interesting food for thought: Women who sleep less than five hours per night are more likely to be overweight and drink more coffee. And we already know that weight alone can lower fertility by up to 50%. So, get out those eye masks, ladies! Lack of sleep will make you hungrier (I suspect as our body craves more energy and looks for it in the wrong place) and does whacky things to hormones. It can even lead to reduced mucus production—not great for fertility.

Men are just as much in need of quality sleep. Their fertility (specifically sperm quality) is affected through testosterone levels, which suffer if they do not get enough shut-eye. Undoubtedly men feel just as awful as a woman do without adequate rest—and are equally as prone to the corresponding weight gain—which in turn affects fertility. Men who are fatigued also have a lower libido and are more likely to experience erectile dysfunction.

Sleep is the elixir of health.

If you aren't sleeping well, it's time to work out why. Allow your health practitioner to guide you towards a better night's sleep. Acupuncture is also fabulous to help relax the body and promote sleep.

You are the best judge of how you are feeling. Nobody can tell you how you feel, so start listening and get in touch with yourself.

❸ Alcohol

This is an interesting topic because the experts are always changing their minds. For one thing, science can't tell us exactly what quantity of alcohol affects fertility, because no two people are the same. But we do know that alcohol consumption definitely decreases reproductive potential. Alcoholic beverages contain oestrogen-like compounds—these 'fake' hormones wreak havoc on our system.

Alcohol substantially lowers zinc absorption—bad news for semen. Lower zinc = less sperm = reduced fertility.

Alcohol has a zapping effect on female hormones, affecting ovulation and menstruation—due to the oestrogen-mimicking properties. For my clients, I suggest low consumption—and for women that's two glasses per week. Anything more than two glasses per week is considered moderate consumption, believe it or not! Many of us would be having more than that on an average Saturday night.

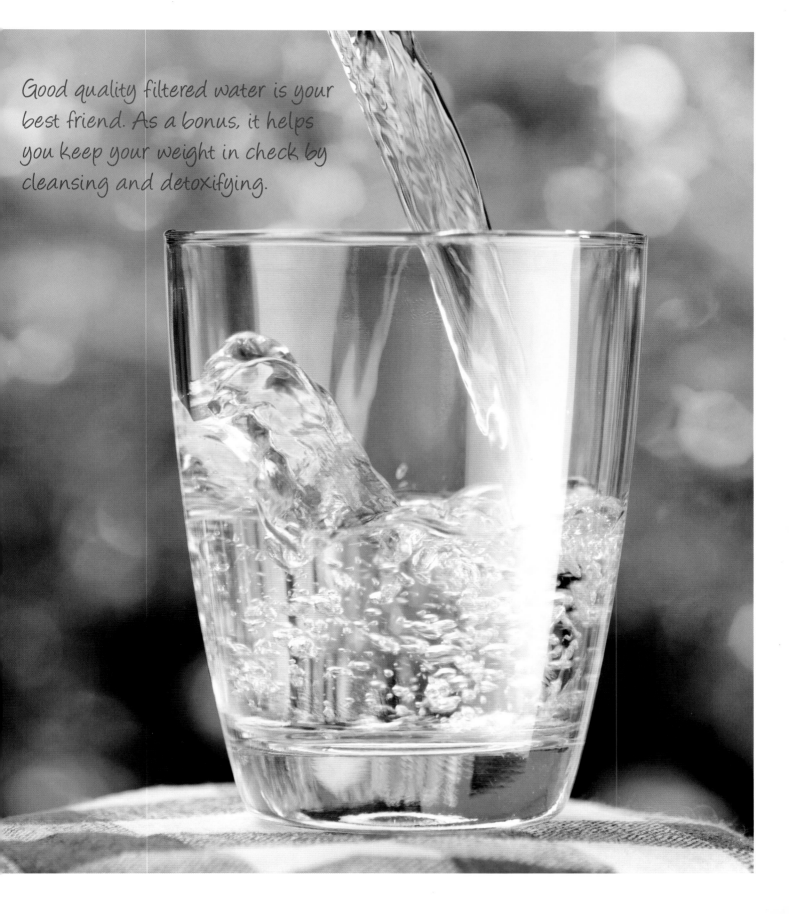

Good quality filtered water is your best friend. As a bonus, it helps you keep your weight in check by cleansing and detoxifying.

Men have a slightly higher tolerance to alcohol, but they should still be very mindful of what they are drinking. Men should aim to have an alcohol-free day every second day and no more than three drinks in a sitting. Mixed drinks can be full of sugar, so switch to a glass of wine or mix with soda.

Moderate to high alcohol consumption has been linked with higher rates of miscarriage. Again, this has to do with its effect on the hormones that are necessary to support pregnancy—particularly progesterone, which is very important in the later stages of the cycle, and human chorionic gonadotropin hormone. Without these, a pregnancy will fail.

❹ Tobacco

If you are a smoker, it's time to say goodbye to the fags. Smoking severely impacts fertility and has been linked to miscarriage. There is not one benefit from smoking, and if you say it de-stresses you, I say find another way to de-stress. Smoking is toxic and, as we now know: a toxic body is not a fertile body.

Perhaps you have fallen into the trap of smoking instead of eating? This robs your body of nutrients in two ways. Eating less obviously equals fewer nutrients, but your body also uses up its vitamin and mineral stores to recover from the toxin hit after every single cigarette you smoke.

Wanting a baby may be more than enough incentive to stop smoking. Aim to quit cold turkey—if you are ready, you can do it. If you're struggling, hypnotherapy can be a wonderful way to say goodbye to unhealthy ways.

Smoking is an absolute no no.

⑤ Exercise

It's simple. You need to move. It doesn't necessarily need to be intense; in fact, intense excercise can do whacky things to ovulation. Just twenty minutes every other day is the perfect amount. Want to do more? That's fine, just be mindful not to overdo it. More than one hour per day can have adverse effects.

Exercise is also important to help to move cortisol (the hormone that occurs in response to stress) through the body.

Gentle exercise like yoga, Pilates and walking are all wonderful ways to get moving. Enjoy lifting weights? Fine, just think a little lighter. Avoid lifting mega-heavy weights.

When cortisol sits in your system, it can set the body into toxic overdrive.

⑥ Water

Get used to purified, good-quality water. It does amazing things for the body, as it helps to cleanse and move toxins out. Toxic build-up is a big fertility killer! Unless you have a rainwater tank or can be completely sure of the quality of your water source, it is important always to filter your water. In cities, medications can filter into the water supply and are rarely captured by treatments. Particularly worrying is the possible presence of hormones from the pill in tap water, **which we will learn can seriously impact your health and fertility.**

Be sure to use a quality filtration system—they aren't expensive. You can purchase jugs that sit on your bench for around $40. I currently have a Bobble filter sitting on my kitchen bench. I love it!

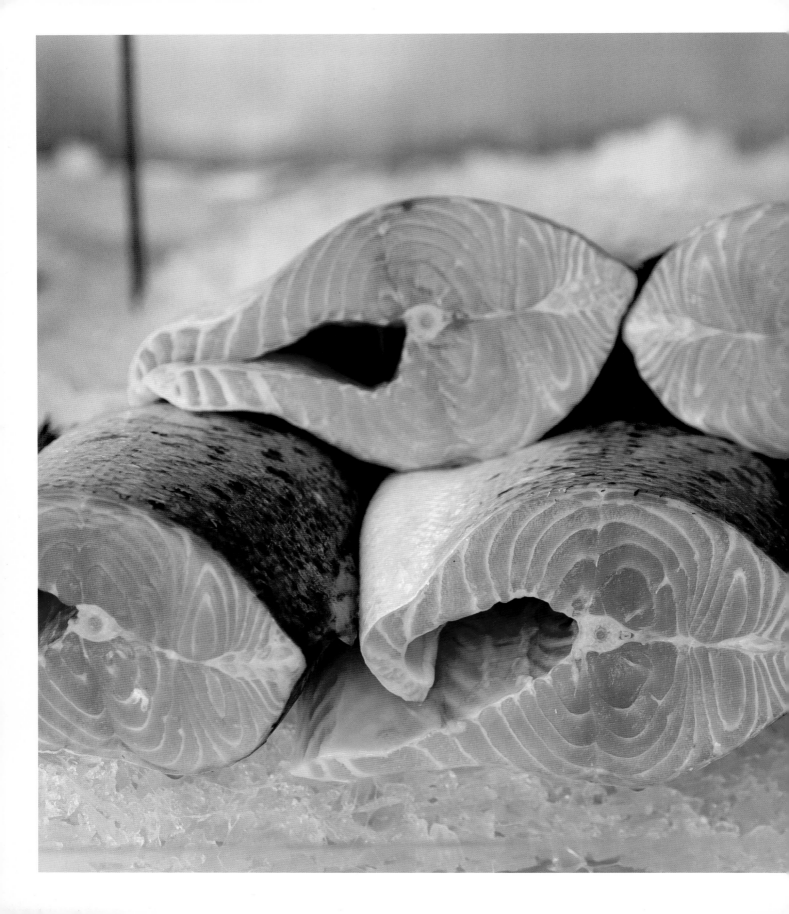

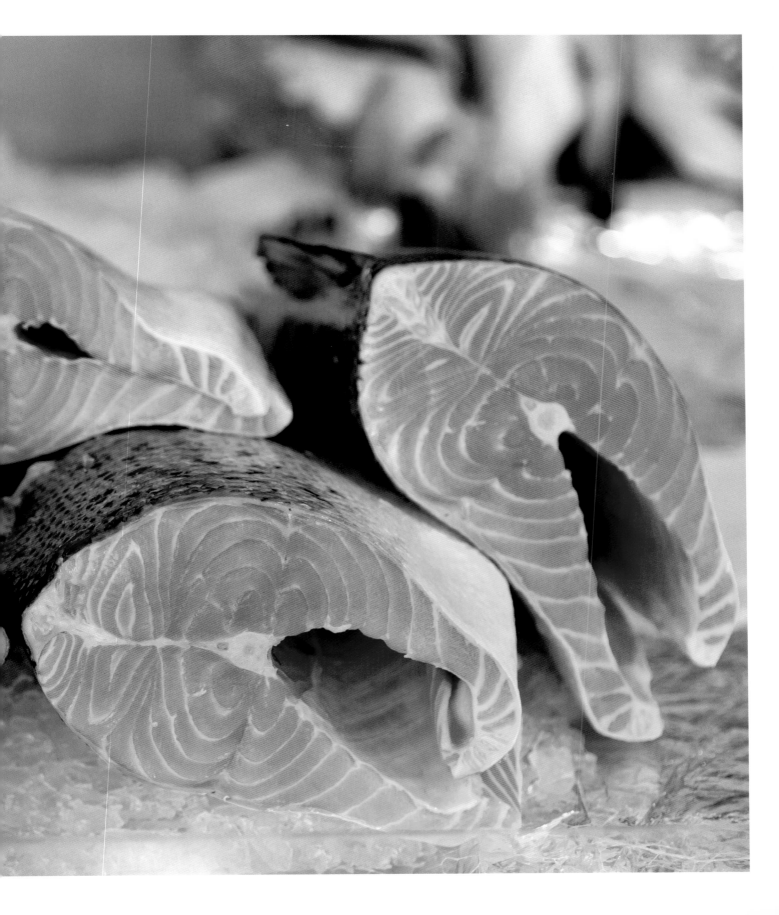

⑦ Emotional Health

Stress decreases fertility by up to 50%. We have already learnt how emotions play a role in overall health, specifically in relation to IVF treatment. Natural conception is no different.

Get happy and healthy—not just for your fertility, but for your overall wellbeing.

⑧ Regular Sex

How much sex do you need to make a baby? Many of my patients will share their anguish over 'baby-making sex'. You know the kind—all about the prize not the ride! The kind that starts off okay, but quickly turns into that hurry-up-and-get-it-over-with-it's-the-third-time-in-three-days-and-I'm-OVER-it! kind of sex.

The biggest mistake I see couples make in the natural fertility game is to confine their timing to what they believe is their ovulatory window. This can be a trap for several reasons.

First, we don't all ovulate at the same time. Forget what your Year 8 teacher taught you in sex ed. Ovulation does not necessarily occur on the fourteenth day of the cycle. The timing of ovulation can be quite elusive, which explains how people so often miss the boat. Second, limiting the amount of intimate time we spend restricts the amount of exercise our reproductive organs receive. An athlete doesn't limit their training to one day a month and, really, neither should your reproductive system.

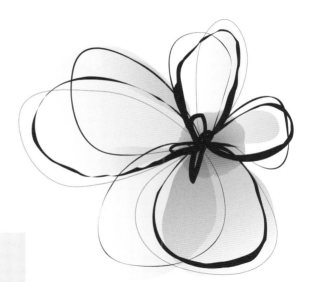

For the Men!

Men who have issues with their semen benefit most from regular sex (when I mention this in the presence of my male clients, they will often feel the need to jump across a room to thank me). I can't remember the last time I saw a good initial semen analysis, and one of the primary aspects of treatment for abnormal and sluggish sperm is plenty of sex.

Abnormal and sluggish sperm needs to be shipped on out to make way for the new and great quality semen we have been working hard to regenerate.

It often takes my male clients up to four months to get semen up to scratch, which suggests to me that nobody can have too much sex for sperm quality and quantity. Many have been led to believe they need to 'save it up', so that the quality will be best during the ovulatory window. But it's not the case! The more frequently you ejaculate, the more room you make for more!

Being busy between the sheets is one of the best ways to improve your sperm and see the quickest change in results. While men generally have a higher libido than women, those with semen issues often do not. By adding regular bedroom activity, we can also see a shift—the more you get the more you want—see how I keep everybody happy! Couples in IVF are advised to pay special attention to semen quality—the better the numbers, the better your chances of success.

A good hug can release hormones that will help you feel good and relieve anxiety and emotional stress ... all in a few seconds!

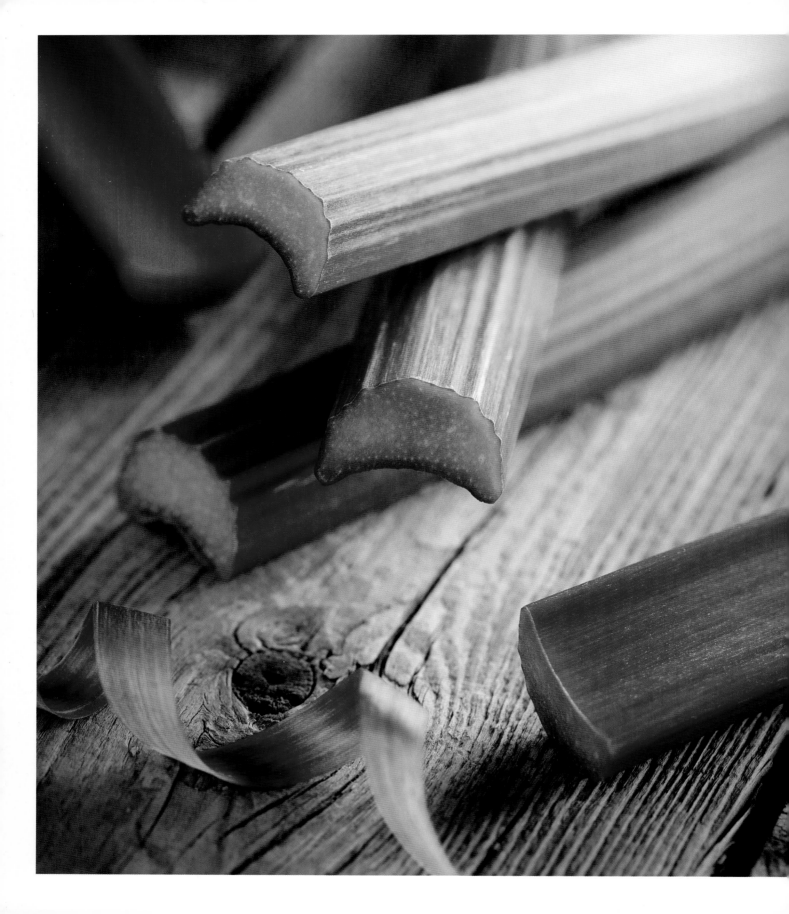

It needs all the exercise it can get to win the baby-making race. This means exercising all month in order to increase blood flow to the female pelvic cavity and to condition and prepare the reproductive area.

By increasing blood flow, we are nourishing the area with all it requires to work best. If a woman has already ovulated and conceived, intercourse in the later part of the cycle will be essential to help the growing embryo embed into the endometrium. This is especially relevant to couples going through IVF. The reproductive organs should be getting all the oxygen and blood supply you can give them.

Women who experience period pain can also benefit from this practice. Increasing activity through the lower abdomen can be a wonderful period-pain cure.

Many of us shudder at the thought of switching off the phone and the TV and stepping away from the laptop, because we just wouldn't know what to do with ourselves (I'm guilty too). And because of all these demands, we rush through dinner and collapse into bed. Add 'time to make a baby' to the schedule and it's just about enough to make you start feeling crazy! It just adds to the stress of the daily routine.

Everyday stresses contribute to lower fertility levels. It's a vicious cycle. So let's just come back to the idea of sex again. Let's just remove the 'baby making' pressure altogether, because we know it crushes intimacy. How about having intimate time as a couple? How about getting back into the practice of regular intimacy between two people who love each other? What about regular sex, just because?! What about no TV or internet in exchange for an early night spent under the covers? That's the

Stress is a modern-day epidemic that we're not necessarily equipped to manage. Becoming aware of your triggers is the first step in overcoming the burden of stress.

A simple dance around the office can be enough to switch on more energy and clear stress. Your colleagues might just join in on the fun!

kind of sex that makes babies. The unplanned, loving, intimate time a couple spend together with one purpose—of just enjoying each other.

Once the baby comes a long, you'll have all the time in the world to worry about the child. But coming back to the original question—how much sex do you need to make a baby? Well, not all that much. But how much sex do you need to be healthy? How much do you need to be physically and mentally nourished? The answer is—lots.

⑨ Know your body

Listen to what your body is saying to you. It speaks to you every day. If you're not getting the messages—ask somebody to help you! Chinese medicine practitioners, nutritionists, herbalists, naturopaths and natural fertility specialists are there to help.

⑩ Sunshine

Sun rays on our skin activate the generation of vitamin D, releasing it into the endocrine system, which drives hormone production. Hormones increase blood flow through the body, increasing oxygen to the brain. And then, what do you know, you feel awesome! And the effects are not limited to feeling good; vitamin D assists with ovulation—so add some sun to your regimen.

In recent years, so much as mention tanning and you can be sent to the naughty spot. With so many campaigns reinforcing the dangers of sun time, we've created a huge health problem. We are designed to soak in some sun. Without it we can get really sick.

The vitamin D that we get from the sun is essential to healthy body function—and fertility.

Finally, health authorities are acknowledging their mistake and have started to re-educate us about just how vital it is to have sun exposure. Sun exposure alone doesn't cause skin cancer. There are many factors that go into the mix of cancer formation: environment, diet, lifestyle, stress, as well as our genetic disposition. I believe that you can set yourself up for optimum health by adding a little sunshine to your day and exposing yourself responsibly.

As a guide, fifteen minutes of unprotected exposure every second day is all you need. Of course, lying out in the sun until you are as crisp as a potato chip doesn't fall into the category of responsible! Be smart. Also watch out for the sunscreen you're wearing—some chemical sunscreens could actually be adding to the skin cancer problem. Where possible, go for natural, physical sunscreens, like zinc-based ones. The ingredients are non-toxic and won't affect your health.

Vitamin D is the kicker of hormone-balancing supplements! It's a must for hormone regulation, mood management and immunity. You can get small amounts from fish and eggs, but your best source is 15 minutes of sun exposure every other day.

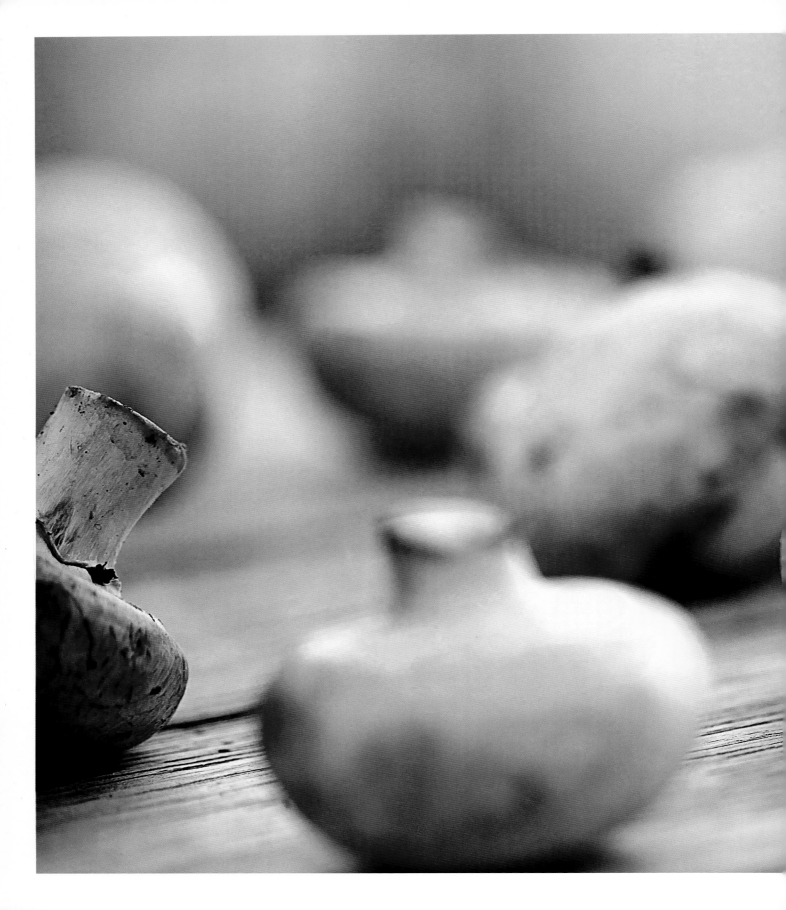

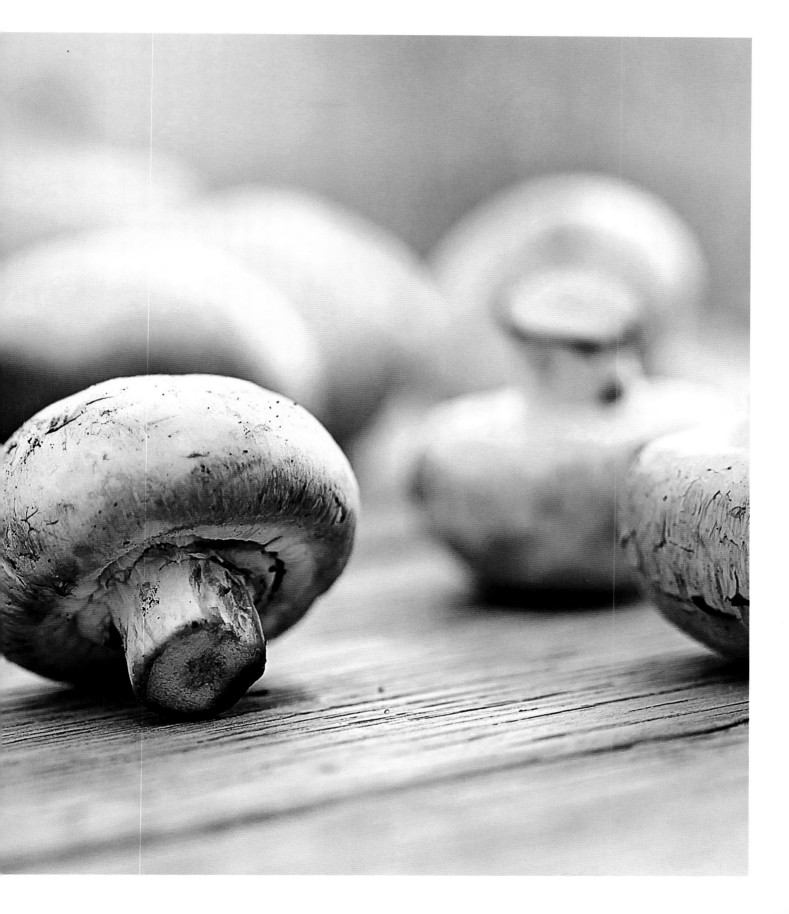

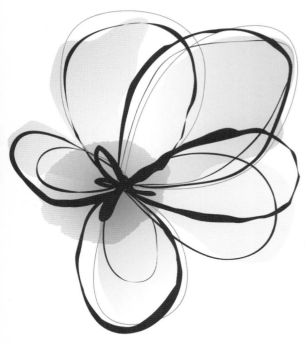

The Drill Down on Hormones

Gut Health: The Pivot of Wellness

As I've made clear, gut health is imperative not only for hormone health but for all-round wellness. I'd like to help you understand this on a deeper level—once you have an understanding you can't help but want to care for your main health centre.

The gut has been likened to a second brain. It's an intricate system that begins in your mouth and extends right through … yeah. Once upon a time, when we were in loincloths, our guts were very well cared for, mostly because our diet supported wellness. Then came refined foods, large-scale agriculture, fridges, fast food, packaging and so on, and we've lost touch with what is actually beneficial for our digestion. As I mentioned earlier, our ancestors knew this intuitively—because their 'guts' told them so.

Your gut is not only the engine of digestion, it is also your emotional centre.

The gut helps us make good decisions based on how we feel—food choices included! In a healthy gut around three litres of bacteria will live happily, ensuring your immunity, digestion, assimilation and defecation is one harmonious symphony.

Gut health is shaped from a very early age—in fact, the gut health of the mother at the time of conception is exactly what the child will inherit. A good dose of probiotics (beneficial bacteria) is delivered through the birth canal during labour as well as through early breast milk, which is also nutrient rich and packed full of antibiotic properties. Long term, breast milk also continues to deliver and balance the gut bacteria as the little one's own digestive system begins to fire up.

Imagine, if you will, a big hose, representing your gut. Now imagine it is lined with a thick protective film on the inside. This represents your gut lining. This lining forms a barrier that keeps your food moving through the gut. When this lining is inflamed or damaged, it prevents the gut doing its job. Inflammatory foods, including refined sugars and gluten, lead to small tears forming in the actual gut wall. Much like a cut on your hand, these tears become irritated and inflamed and allow food to escape the system. This leakage then becomes toxic, as it leeches somewhere in the body it isn't supposed to be. This is a condition commonly known as leaky gut and it can cause a host of conditions, including hormone imbalance, allergies, digestive troubles and irritable bowel syndrome (a blanket name for a host of symptoms).

Modern lifestyles mean that in most people, gut health is poor. Medications, poor dietary habits, lifestyle, stress and emotional turmoil all compromise delicate gut bacteria, and key strains of bacteria are often missing. To compound this, babies are formula fed and sometimes too freely given antibiotics, both of which hinder the early growth of healthy gut bacteria. If no action is taken by the unwell adult to restore

The gut has been likened to a second brain—it helps control many of the body's functions, including your emotions. That's why people who suffer from anxiety and emotional disorders notice vast improvements when they give their digestive system some TLC.

Eat consciously.
You will love yourself for it.

the gut, illness and sometimes long-term health problems can develop.

My hope is that the community at large will get on board the fix-your-gut bandwagon. In previous times, probiotic and fermented foods were part of the daily diet, largely because in the days before refrigeration preserving foods through fermentation was one of the only means of surviving periods of short supply. Whether or not our forbears knew how healthy fermented foods are is irrelevant—they had found the secret to replenishing and restoring healthy gut flora.

Nowadays there are many things that will upset the beautiful digestive balance.

The overuse of medications—especially the pill and antibiotics—is one of the major causes in gut ill health. Just as the name suggests, antibiotics will kill gut flora. Antibiotics are a genius idea—as long as you don't think about it too much. The problem with antibiotics is, if you wipe out all bacteria, you're knocking out the good, balancing and nourishing bacteria with the bad ones. It doesn't take long to clear them out, but it can take years of care to restore them. Some essential bacteria will never grow back after a dose of antibiotics—our bodies don't just grow more, like a strand of hair or a pinkie nail do. Some vital bacteria can take up to sixteen months to fully grow back with the help of probiotics and fermented foods. Doctors don't tell us about these drawbacks, which is

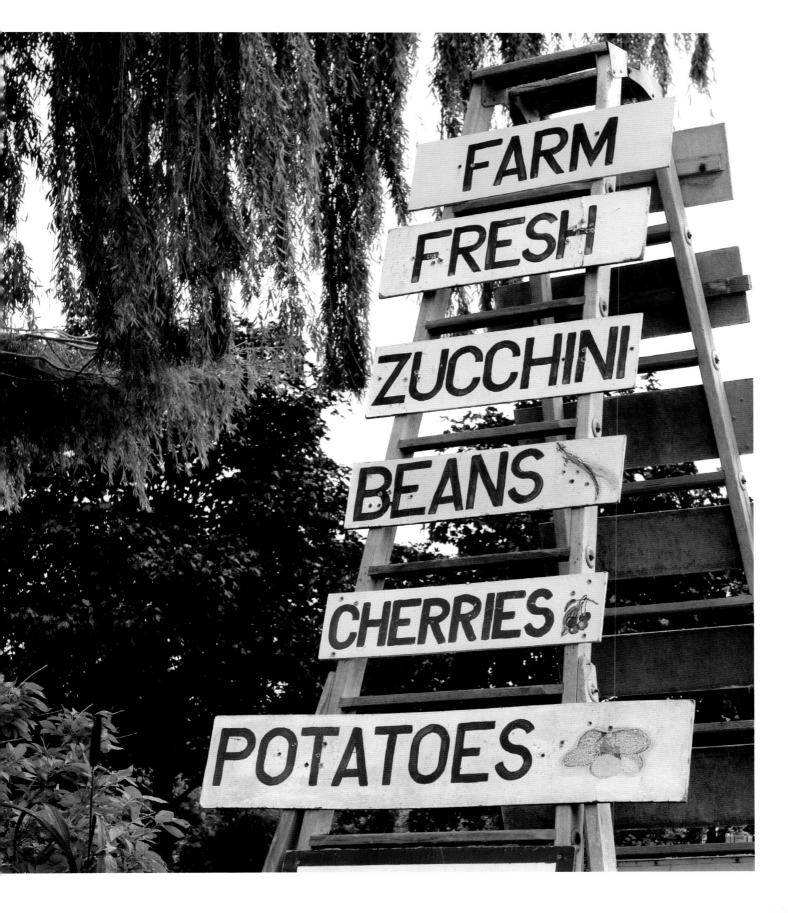

why we will readily accept antibiotics in situations that don't actually warrant them or could even make our situation worse, given that gut health influences our immune health too.

We've seemingly lost faith in our bodies when we fall ill. In most instances, under the right circumstances our bodies have the ability to heal, but we've been conditioned to think otherwise. We're so quick to reach into the medicine cabinet, but stopping to think about the cause of the illness helps us to put things into perspective—is it just part of a process? Consider a flu. We're mad for a dose of paracetamol to bring the thermometer reading down. But the fever is part of the body's natural response in the process of healing an illness. Raising the temperature helps the body to open the pores and sweat out the 'bug'. Perhaps you've taken paracetamol and noticed that your fever is gone, but you still feel lousy and the flu continues to last for several days. The breaking of the fever is the turning point of the illness—if we interfere, the illness is going to last longer because the body never gets the chance to fully go through the motions of recovery.

Your body is actually pretty intelligent—every symptom has a function, and, if we give it a chance, we have the ability to recover pretty quickly. Gut health is an integral part of allowing your body to heal naturally.

'The days you are most uncomfortable are the days you learn the most about yourself.'

LORNA JANE

So how can you get your gut in good condition?

First, we must restore the delicate bacterial balance, remembering that it takes time. By eating fermented foods and probiotics like kombucha, sauerkraut and pickled veggies, as well as kefir and yoghurt, we can begin to restore gut flora. The lifestyle choices I discuss in this book are all equally important. We need to eat less man-made, processed foods and more whole foods and superfoods. We can take all the probiotics and multivitamins on the planet, but if we continue to eat sugar and gluten, the gut will not heal. And as we know, gut health is key to happy hormones.

Let's not forget that the pill is a method of contraception and simply can't cure hormone imbalances.

The Pill

The pill was never designed to be a treatment. It was developed as a contraception method to prevent pregnancy.

The pill is now the most prescribed drug worldwide.

The problem is, the pill severely depletes wellness. It strips the gut of essential bacteria, which causes the body to stop absorbing the vitamins and minerals from food and drink. Your body then dips into its stores of these vitamins and minerals, using up your reserve tank. Because the tank isn't being topped up, many women find themselves severely affected by the pill. Even if you're not seeing side effects, the pill may still be affecting you.

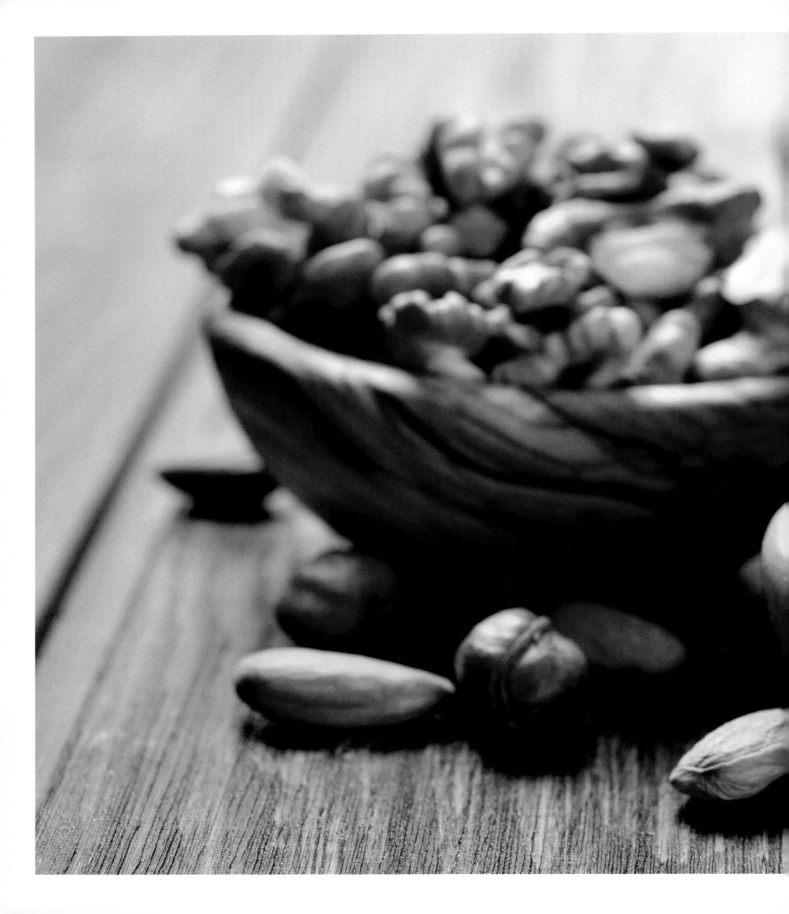

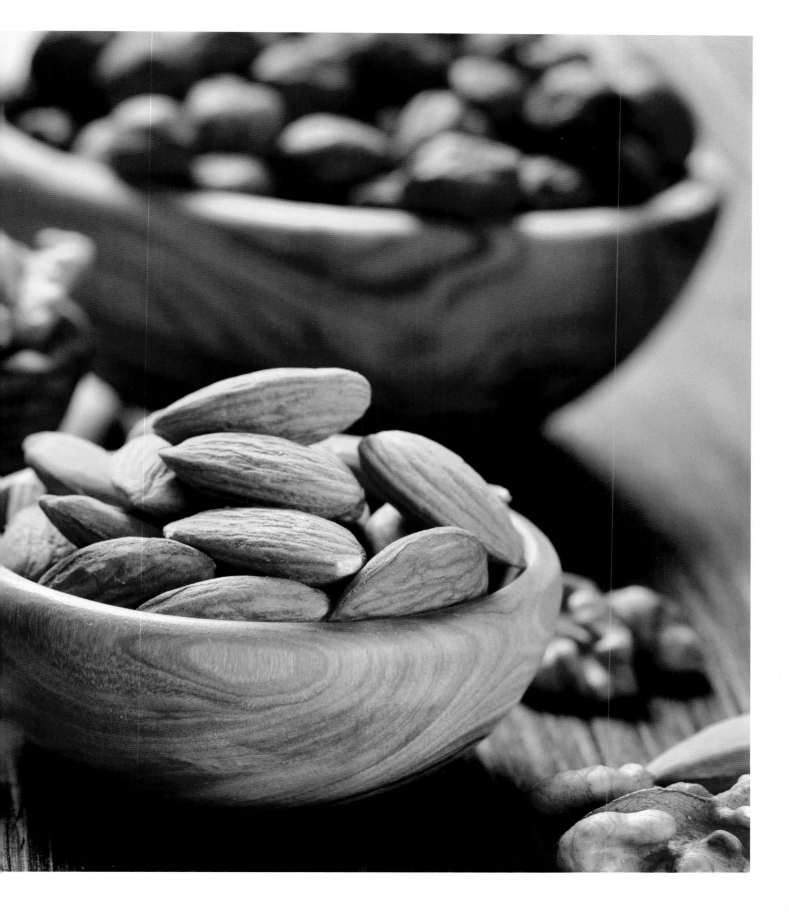

Close your eyes and imagine the best version of yourself—that's who you are. Now just go and make it happen.

If your body is speaking to you by way of acne, painful periods, PMS, amenorrhea (missing periods), PCOS or endometriosis, the pill is not a long-term solution, because it doesn't treat the root cause of the condition. The only true way to heal is to get to the crux of the matter. It's more than likely your GP has been led to believe that the pill is a safe option and it will treat your hormone imbalance. But sadly, the pill cannot cure hormone imbalance because it covers up the real issue.

For some women, taking the pill is wonderful, and easy contraception provides a huge sense of relief. But at what cost? It's important that the message about the long-term ramifications of taking the pill gets out, especially while fourteen-year-old girls are regularly prescribed the pill for acne or PMS.

Many women report that they feel crazy while on the pill; they have mood swings, low libido, headaches and break-through bleeding, and they feel fuzzy and generally off. What a fantastic contraception method! With this mixed bag of symptoms, I have to ask, who'd want sex anyway? Apart from the side effects, another issue is that many young girls (and women) are less likely to use condoms, which would normally protect them from a range of sexually transmitted diseases (STDs) and pelvic inflammatory disorders (PIDs).

PIDs are a big deal for women, as they can cause long-term damage to the reproductive organs. To think that a fourteen-year-old girl is responsible enough to take the pill daily is ambitious to say the least (I remember being fourteen—I knew better than the prime minister!). The pill prevents girls from getting to know their bodies by reading the signs and symptoms of the cycle. And it is causing them further health problems.

As I mentioned earlier, the pill is contributing to our collective gut health issues. The pill, just like antibiotics, clears out vital, good bacteria from the gut. For this reason, the long-term effects of the pill are said to spread across three generations. As we've learnt, at the time of conception the mother directly passes on her gut health to her baby, so if the mother is compromised, the baby will inherit an incomplete set of bacteria. If the child, once grown up, never acts on restoring its gut health, it too will pass on its poor health.

Perhaps you've chosen to take the pill or you've been taking it with the belief that it is preventing much more than a baby (we're told it reduces the risk of ovarian cancer, saves our bones, treats endometriosis, PCOS, acne—the works). I'd encourage you to look to treating the cause instead, and of course the diet and lifestyle tricks outlined in this book are your best starting point. Gut repair and ultimate health are absolute musts for happy hormone health.

Your body communicates through nerves and hormones. Make sure it's firing all the right signals, otherwise you'll find hair in places it doesn't belong or perhaps the appetite of a sumo wrestler. Either way, it isn't pretty.

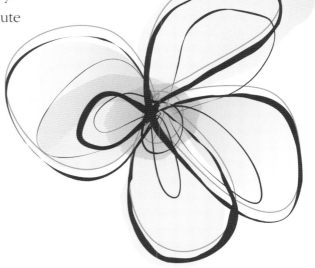

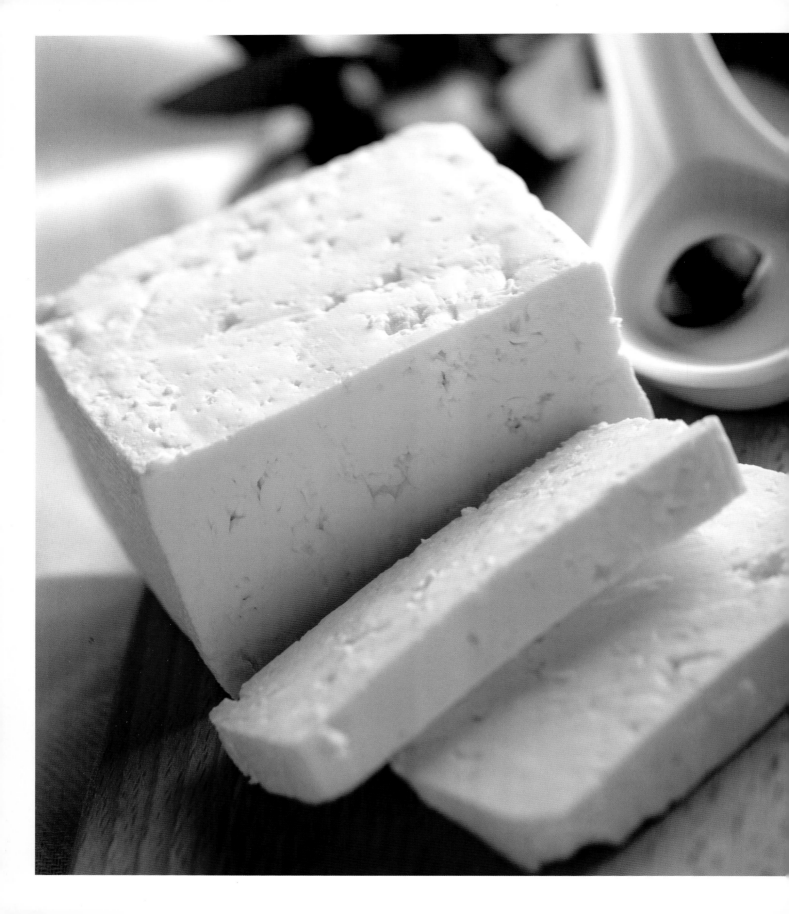

Pre Fertility: Revving It Up!

No matter your situation, it is imperative that you reach your maximum wellness before conception. Of course, babies are conceived in all kinds of scenarios, sometimes without planning, and that's perfectly okay—many of us wouldn't be here otherwise. But if you have decided to conceive then it's time to focus on wellness and fertility. We're not living in the same world our parents did. Food quality is different, stress is much higher and couples are having babies later: these all impact our fertility. The bottom line is this: our bodies need a certain level of health if we want to conceive with ease— whether through IVF or assisted conception, or just the natural way.

It all begins with awareness. Gaining knowledge about your body helps you make decisions that are right for your unique self.

Without certain nuts and bolts, a car won't run. Your body is no different. If your menstrual cycle is all over the shop or your period is missing, your body is telling you something—you can't skimp on health. If your body is deficient, chances are you'll have trouble conceiving. Especially for couples facing IVF, health is without doubt the most important piece of the puzzle.

If you think western medicine will save you if natural fertility fails, think again. The odds are not great.

Let's look at clomifene (Clomid). I'm not opposed to it, but it is problematic. If you're not familiar with clomifene, it is a drug that promotes ovulation. Basically, it works by blocking the action of oestrogen so that the pituitary gland is tricked into producing lots of follicle-stimulating hormone (FSH). It's freely prescribed, most often to women who are still having trouble conceiving after a period of around six months.

Some doctors will be thorough enough to run blood tests before prescribing clomifene to check whether a woman is actually ovulating—the blood sample is typically taken on the twenty-first day of the cycle. The doctor then works out a treatment plan according to the result. But here's the problem: what if ovulation happens after the twenty-first of the cycle? Most likely, the patient will be told she isn't ovulating and will be prescribed Clomid, even though she might well be ovulating! The Debunking Ovulation section later covers how a woman can know if she is ovulating or not without blood tests or invasive methods. Not everything is as straightforward as medical science would have it. A blood test provides only a snapshot of a short period of time, not the full picture.

From a natural fertility viewpoint, the benefit that clomifene offers (promoting ovulation) is cancelled out by all that it robs from your body. Most importantly, it reduces fertile mucus (essential for conception) and thins the uterus lining, making the environment unfavourable for conception. The success rates for clomifene are low, and each time the clomifene course is repeated the unwanted side effects compound the problem. Other side effects of clomifene include enlarged ovaries, irritability, headaches, nausea, vomiting and more.

But for a very few, clomifene can be fantastic, especially if hormone health and wellness are being nurtured—keep in

Maximising your health—no matter what your situation is—can only lead to an improved state of all-round wellness. Thinking that our bodies will adjust without making changes isn't logical. To create change, we must do something differently.

mind it only works for those who aren't ovulating. Often, the anguish of trying unsuccessfully for a baby long-term takes its toll. Emotional stress is on par with physical stress in terms of its effect on hormone balance.

So how do we pump up the fertile factor? My advice is always the same, whether for general hormone balance, PCOS, endometriosis or thyroid issues. By putting my diet and lifestyle guidelines in place and decreasing stress, you will get to optimum hormone health.

Post Birth: Settling Those Hormones Down

Balancing hormones and making babies is the fun part. On the other side of pregnancy, flourishing hormones will be quite a different experience, often stranger than anything else we experience in our lives as women.

A hormone known as relaxin, which makes its debut during the later stages of pregnancy, will continue to be present for up to five months post birth. This is the hormone responsible for making things stretch. Your body, specifically your muscles, becomes more supple in preparation for birth. Women often find their joints to be loose or easily injured post birth, and relaxin is the reason. Relaxin makes us relax.

Now, as you know, your body's signs and symptoms are communicating with you. Prolactin is the hormone that causes milk production, and it is also an appetite stimulant. It's important to be mindful that it's normal to feel hungry and eating

Giving birth is no mean feat! Reward yourself by allowing yourself time to recover and fall in love with your new little family!

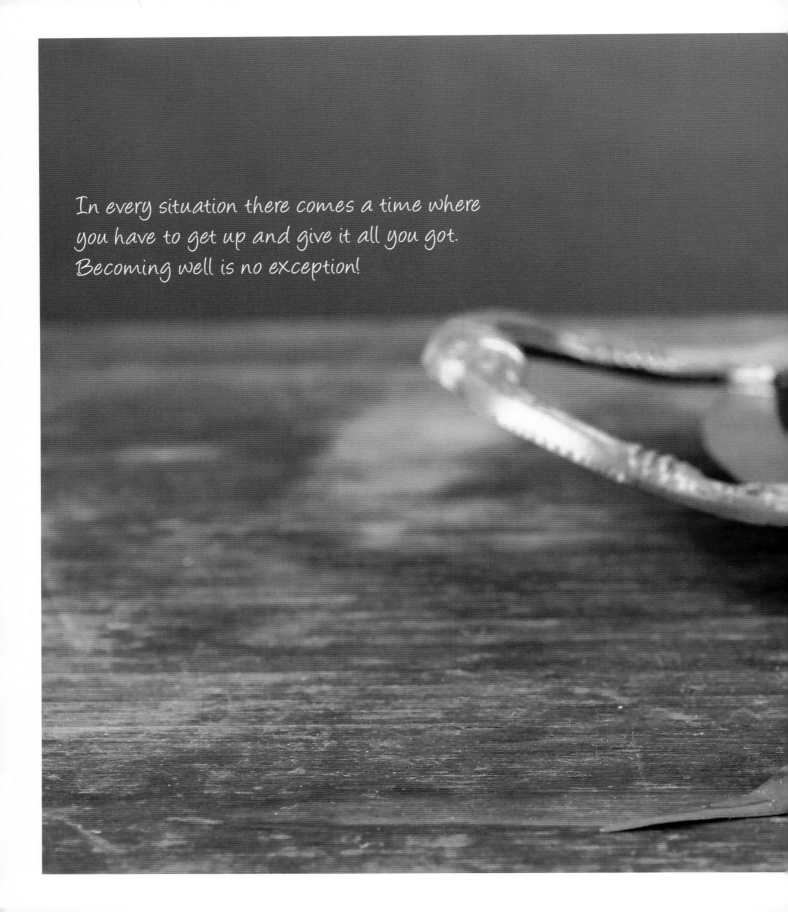

In every situation there comes a time where
you have to get up and give it all you got.
Becoming well is no exception!

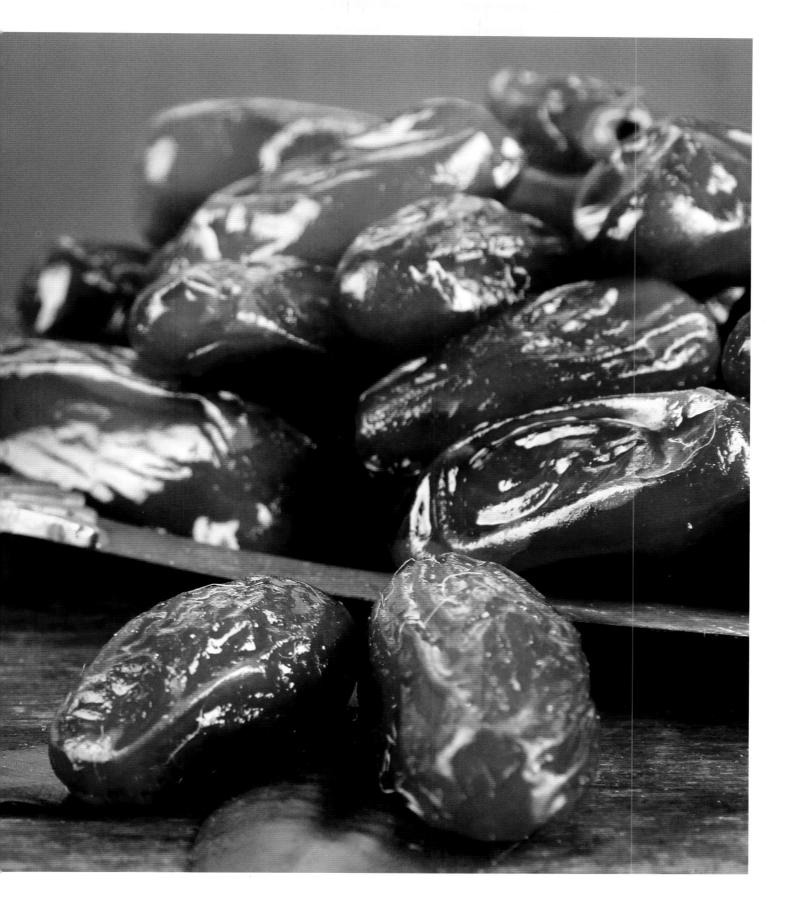

according to your body's commands is vital for your milk supply. Not only does your baby inherit your gut health, but it also gets an almighty dose of probiotics on the way out of the birth canal. The icing on the cake is breastfeeding, which also contains antibodies that are beneficial for gut health and nourishment. This package lays the best foundation, in a perfect world.

After having a baby, women often find themselves ravenously hungry.

If your body is well prepared and cared for before and during your pregnancy, there is less chance that you will come crashing down when your baby is born.

Not all of us are fortunate enough to experience a vaginal delivery, nor do some people wish to. I was fortunate enough (at least for my clients) to experience both; a natural, drug-free birth with my daughter and then a c-section with all the trimmings in the drug department with my son. The latter, while not my choice, has helped me understand more about the flipside, especially relating to gut health. I knew I had to ensure my son was getting all the good bacteria possible to make up for what he didn't receive upon arrival into this big, beautiful world. Those probiotics I mentioned earlier are essential for babies—whether through breast milk or otherwise, it's important our children have these from a young age for optimal wellness.

Hormone levels drop immediately after birth because the placenta is the major source of hormone production through the later stages of pregnancy. Every woman has a different response to this drop—but if your body is well prepared and cared for pre-pregnancy and during it, there is less chance that you will come crashing down post birth.

One of the most noticeable changes after birth can be in mood. This is simply due to the rapid decline in hormones. Planning ahead to pep yourself up is a good idea. To think we can survive on our own without support or help is madness. In many cultures, women are put on bed rest or set themselves up at home and don't leave for a period of time (typically around forty days). Before having children I thought that was rather luxurious. After having two myself and studying Chinese medicine in-depth, I now know that birth is a massive event your body needs to recover from, and you also have a newborn baby to adjust to and care for. We can't all get help twenty-four/seven, but it is important to be mindful that we aren't actually designed to do it on our own. We need help and support so we can recover and nurture our newborn baby.

We now understand that the gut is our second brain and our emotional centre and we know that vital gut bacteria shapes overall wellness. If this delicate environment is upset, the body won't absorb the nutrients from food that fuel the body's functions—including producing hormones. If we have our gut department covered, there is far less chance postnatal depression will take hold beyond the expected, short-term baby blues.

The secret to kicking the baby blues is in having a strong and healthy gut. Nourishing yourself and your baby is paramount for happy healthy hormones.

One of the most commonly misunderstood post-birth conditions is postnatal depression.

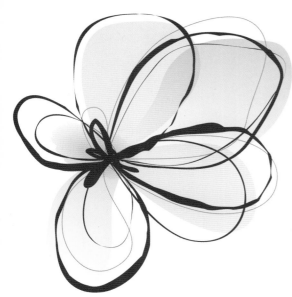

It is normal to feel overwhelmed and even experience sadness post birth as the hormone levels plummet. The secret to kicking the blues lies within a strong and healthy gut. Eating probiotic foods daily is a must for everyone, pregnant or not. Children and babies too!

Post Birth Help

Here are a few important tips to help makes those few weeks post birth easier. Read them now —in those blurry few weeks following birth you may have trouble finding the time to read.

WATER Hydrating yourself ensures you are well nourished. And warm baths will help to ease tiredness and soreness.

SALT I'm in love with Peruvian pink salt—it's so healing inside and out. Think of it as your daily mineral dose. Add it to your food, or to your bath to help relaxation and heal any grazes or sore nipples.

MULTIVITAMINS This is the time when your vitamin and mineral stores can plummet. Be sure to take supplements for at least six months after birth. This will also help in fighting postnatal depression.

FISH OIL This is chock full of omega-3 and omega-6, which are both essential for the brain development of your child (through breast milk) and for your emotional wellness, skin nourishment (healing and stretch marks) and general health.

SLEEP! Easier said than done, but it is the elixir of health. Sleep when your baby sleeps—it's not a crime!

BONE BROTH One of the most nourishing and healing foods there is. Because of the cooking process, broth made from meat and bone is full of vitamins and minerals to restore your health.

REST It goes without saying, but as a new mum I needed constant reminding. Your body needs it for recovery and to nurture your new baby! Get in some rest whenever you can.

CALL ON YOUR TRIBE Draw on your little community for support and help. No new mother should begin to entertain the thought she can do it alone. After all, no other species does!

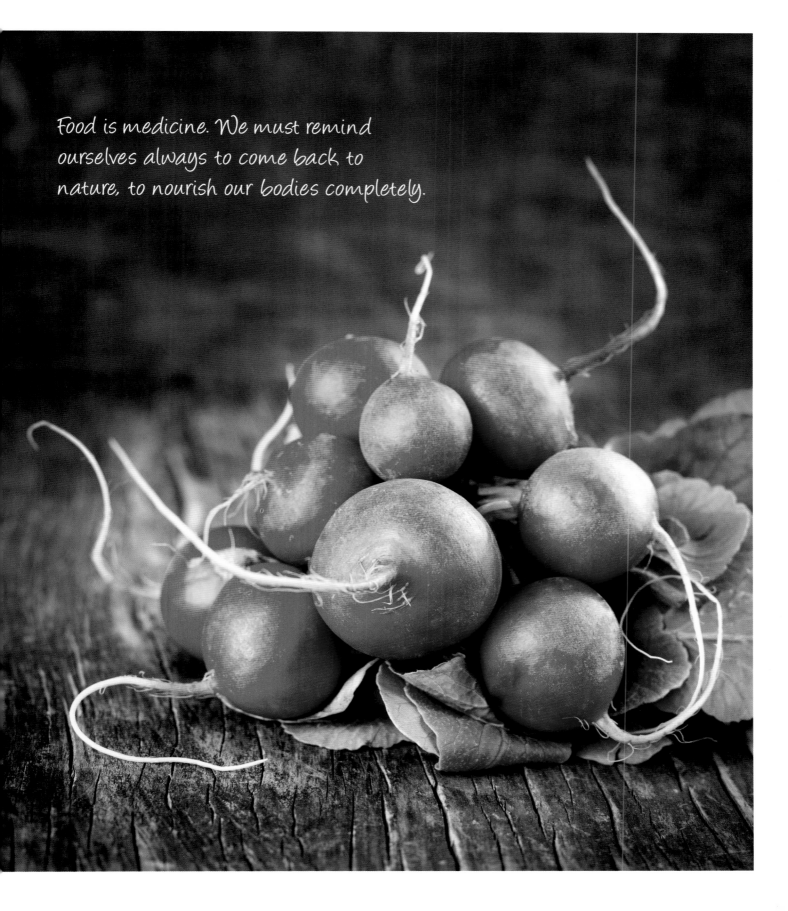

Food is medicine. We must remind
ourselves always to come back to
nature, to nourish our bodies completely.

The weeks post birth can be so confusing. More than anything, remind yourself to come back to nature, by continuing to incorporate proteins and fats at every meal to make sure your body is well supported, and to call on others for help. It will allow you to rest, and I guarantee that your friends and family will love having the chance to help you!

Debunking Ovulation

In many cases what we learnt about our bodies and menstrual cycles in our teen years was far from the truth: we can't fall pregnant all month round, nor do we ovulate on the same day every month.

Think of your laptop or smart phone—all our devices need charging. Through lack of awareness, spending less and less time in social circles and through medications like the pill feeding us synthetic hormones, we have literally stopped charging our bodies. We've pulled the plug. In western culture, we aren't taught to read our body's fertility signals, and we're less likely to talk about our bodily experiences, as we shy away from too much 'girl talk'. So, we don't really that know much about ourselves. What's more, pretty much everything we were taught in sex ed in school was wrong. We were told that we shouldn't have sex because we can fall pregnant just like that, at pretty much any time of the month; that we all collectively ovulate on the fourteenth day of our cycle, and that women must all suffer from period pain. Could these 'facts' be any further from the truth?

We've got so much of this body stuff wrong, and lack of real knowledge causes problems for so many women. Nobody understands your own body better than you can. There are so many variations on the 'normal' cycle, but for clarity I'm going to take it back to how it should look in theory. I want you to understand the table on the next pages thoroughly, so I'm going to break it down to simple town. Remember, it is a rough guide only.

Should your cycle be a bit out of whack—if ovulation is occurring earlier or later than suggested on the chart—your body may be responding to a hormonal imbalance, and the consequence is a state we call sub-fertility. This means that, while you might be fertile, your hormones are in need of adjustment. So, for example, if ovulation happens on day 9 of the cycle something is not right, because an immature follicle is being released—making it almost impossible for it to be fertilised. Or, if your luteal phase (ovulation to the period) is too short an embryo won't be able to grow because it isn't getting all the hormones it requires. In almost all cases, this can be naturally treated, and by following the guidelines in this book you can begin to correct the imbalance.

For a novice, the idea of sensing your way through your menstrual cycle will be a bit strange for the first few months. But reading your body's signs will soon become second nature. Some people successfully use this knowledge of the unique phases of their cycle as a contraceptive method. I encourage those using this method to keep in mind two things. First, from the time we start to notice moistness right through until ovulation is the time we need to be most mindful, and, second, we must count three days from the last wet day to know the fertile phase has passed.

A few other things about your period that I would encourage you to know are these: if you experience a one-day bleed that

You are a product of your environment. Many factors can influence your menstrual cycle—some you might never have thought of.

	DAYS	INFORMATION
1	Period – heavy	Pain
2	Period – medium	
3	Period – medium	
4	Period – light	
5	Spotting	
6	Dry	
7	Dry	
8	Dry	
9	Dry	
10	Moist	
11	Moist	
12	Moist	
13	Wet	
14	Wet	
15	Wet	Ovulation
16	Dry	
17	Dry	
18	Dry	
19	Dry	
20	Dry	
21	Dry	
22	Dry	
23	Dry	
24	Dry	
25	Dry	Tender Breasts
26	Dry	PMS
27	Dry	PMS
28	Dry	PMS and Irritability

Model Cycle

Let's walk through it. The first phase of the cycle is called the follicular phase—from the first day of the period (bleeding) until ovulation. The period can last anywhere between two and seven days. For my clients, I like to see a period of no longer than five days, and if a woman is bleeding beyond this or experiences very heavy and painful periods I will implement strategies to treat this. It is important that blood loss is not too significant— about six tablespoons used to be a good guide, but it is difficult to tell the amount with the current standard of sanitary products.

You will normally experience several 'dry' days before you start to notice a small amount of mucus (days 6–9), followed by a feeling of moistness (days 10–12). This can last for several days until you begin to feel signs of optimal fertility—typically, clear and stretchy cervical mucus. A trick is to notice that during ovulation the opening of the vagina feels wet and cold, although this is often already towards the end of ovulation. This cervical mucus is essential for conception. It is the sperm's mode of transport up to the waiting egg. When the semen is ejaculated into the vagina, it will make its way up to the cervical crypts, where it stays for a bit, to take a little rest, to be fed and rejuvenated (I find it hilarious that it is already hungry!), before it continues on up to meet the egg. If you take a look at fertile cervical mucus under a microscope, it has many little channels—unlike infertile mucus, which has a grid-like pattern that makes it impossible for the sperm to swim through.

In our model cycle, ovulation occurs on day 15, the last wet day, even though fertile mucus has been present for three days prior—as I mentioned, it is normally on the final day that the wet feeling is experienced. At first, when you start noticing these patterns, you probably won't know until after the event, but as you get a better sense for it you'll be able to read your own body rhythms more clearly.

From day 16 right through to day 28 you will notice there is very little or no mucus. During this time (the luteal phase) your body is busy either implanting an embryo if you've timed sex right or preparing for your period. Should you notice mucus or discharge at this time, it may be indicative of excess damp in your body, which may or may not be affecting your fertility. In Chinese medicine, damp is what we refer to when there is an accumulation of moisture in your body, as a result of some organs not working as well as they should. It can be easily fixed.

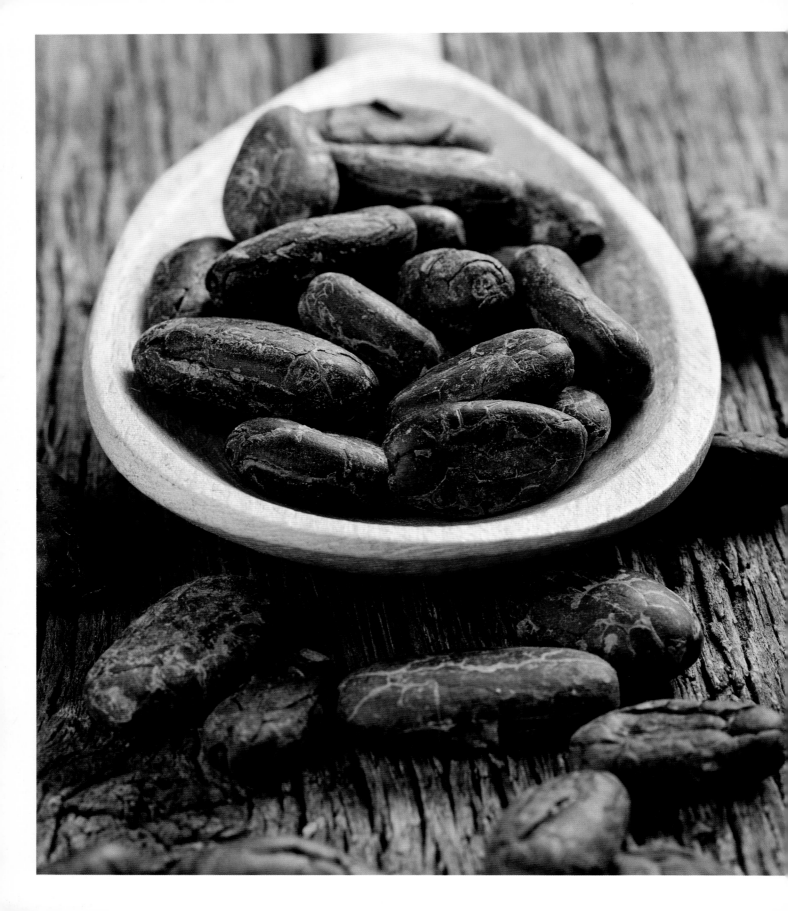

is quite dry and dark without proper flow, there is a chance you aren't ovulating, and it would be a good idea to speak to a natural fertility specialist. And, if you are getting a period with normal bleeding, you are absolutely ovulating—it's just a matter of knowing when. Finally, know this: ovulation will always be followed by a period if you are not pregnant.

Very often women will express their concerns to me that they aren't ovulating, but let me reiterate: if you are getting a period then you are absolutely ovulating. As I've mentioned before, your GP may offer an ovulation test, which is performed on day 21 of the cycle, but you may in fact be ovulating after the twenty-first day of the cycle, so the test method is somewhat flawed.

The Truth about Polycystic Ovarian Syndrome

If you don't have it, I would bet my last dollar that you know somebody who does. Polycystic ovarian syndrome (PCOS) is a result of hormone imbalance—whereby a woman overproduces male hormones (androgens). Typically she presents with two out of three of the following symptoms:

- polycystic ovaries (confirmed by ultrasound)
- blood test or symptoms confirming male hormone presence
- irregular periods (typically fewer than six per year).

When we look at an ultrasound of the ovaries of a woman with PCOS, there will usually be more follicles on the ovaries than in a healthy woman. Normally, as each individual follicle matures, it goes through a series of events that stimulates the hormones that induce ovulation—when a follicle becomes an egg.

The issue for women with PCOS
is that while they have an oversupply of follicles,
these rarely produce eggs capable of being fertilised.

It is estimated that 12–18% of Australian women of reproductive age have PCOS. Symptoms vary, but women with PCOS experience one or more of the following:

- irregular menstrual cycles
- missing periods (amenorrhea)
- acne
- weight gain
- irritability
- anxiety
- depression
- pelvic pain
- skin pigmentation
- weak joints
- weak nails
- thinning hair
- poor gut health
- bowel issues
- facial hair
- sleep apnoea.

Thinking that the contraceptive pill can heal PCOS is like thinking you can fly a unicorn to Mars ...

It's widely accepted that excess androgens may be present in women with the syndrome, which will alter the way their hormones interact. But in the clinic I've begun to see a new wave of PCOS women. They don't technically fit the profile. We're going to dive into why, but before we do, let's look at what causes PCOS.

Why Does PCOS Happen?

Until recently it was thought that insulin resistance was the main factor in PCOS. But it has become clear that it is more complex. Other factors that have been linked to PCOS include synthetic oestrogen (the pill), genetics and environmental factors.

Insulin resistance is absolutely the crux of the issue. Insulin is a hormone secreted by the pancreas in response to rising blood glucose levels (from eating sugary foods, for example). The main function of insulin is to activate the cells to take up glucose so that it isn't roaming around in our blood stream. So imagine your cells are like little sponges, absorbing any excess glucose in your system when insulin gives the order.

Insulin-resistant people require much higher amounts of insulin to be released for their cells to respond. In turn, the system goes a little haywire and produces excess testosterone. This excess testosterone triggers PCOS. This is classic hormone imbalance.

The classic tell-tale symptoms of PCOS are changing. No longer do we see all women with PCOS having facial hair or being overweight. This, too, is a sign that our bodies are changing and we need to understand why.

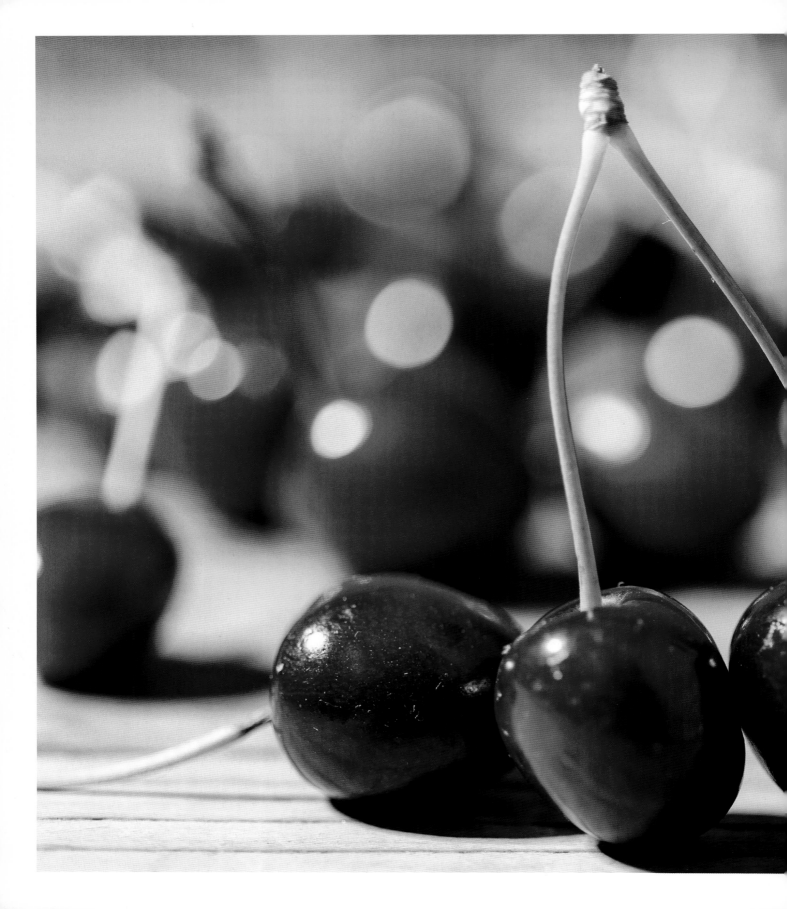

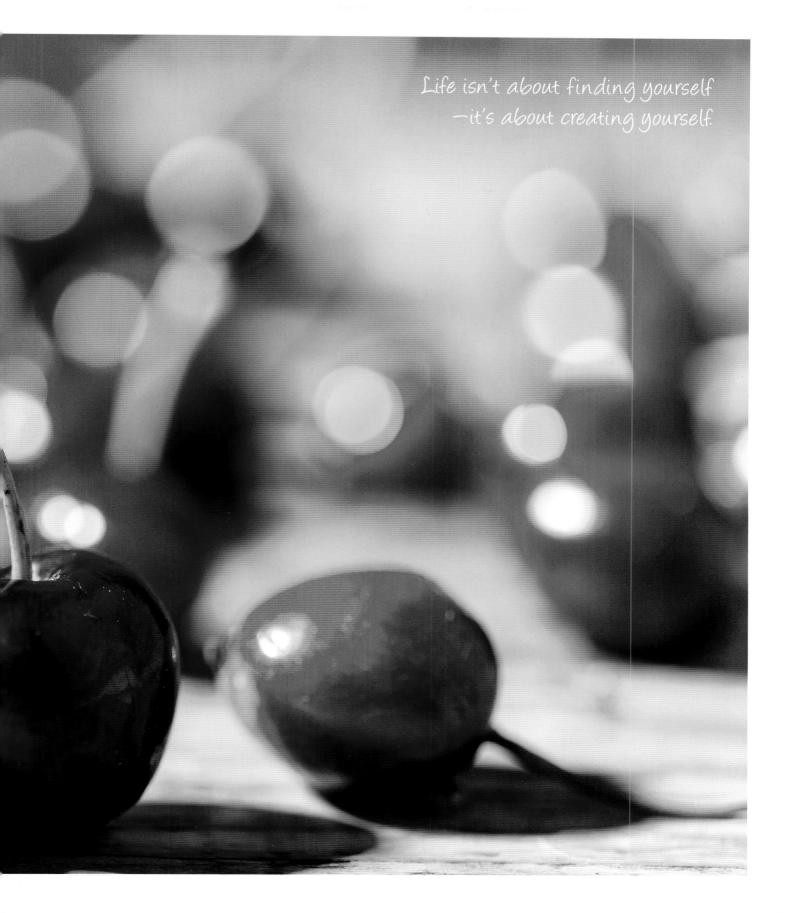

Life isn't about finding yourself
—it's about creating yourself.

Fluctuating sugar levels

Adrenaline release

The liver releases
additional glucose in
expectation of the brain's
requirement for extra fuel

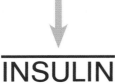

INSULIN

Increased testosterone
due to high levels of
under-utilised insulin.

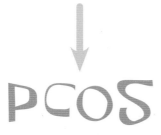

PCOS

In a healthy body insulin acts on the ovary to make testosterone, which is necessary for producing oestrogen. Most women with PCOS have high blood-insulin levels, so their ovaries overproduce testosterone. Rising testosterone levels act as a brake on the menstrual cycle, as well as presenting other unwanted symptoms like facial hair and acne.

The two key factors influencing insulin resistance are diet and weight. Genetic disposition can play a very small role but the key lies in weight control. Unfortunately, women with insulin resistance tend to gain weight easily, which worsens insulin resistance. It is a vicious cycle.

There are several important factors in the treatment of PCOS. I've broken it down to five key points.

1 DIET AND LIFESTYLE These are vital for women with PCOS, as for all women. Undoing the vicious cycle of PCOS sugar cravings starts with following a whole-food diet. Gut health is imperative. If the gut isn't assimilating, we can't readily use the fuel we're putting in, and it gets stored as fat. Food allergies and intolerances will also compromise absorption. If you can't absorb, you can't nourish or heal.

2 MINIMISE STRESS Stress sets off a chain of the events in the body. As shown in the diagram on page 74, it triggers the production of cortisol and adrenaline—stress hormones—which severely disrupt the production of other hormones such as progesterone and serotonin—required for sleep.

Lack of serotonin also causes food cravings and leads to magnesium (required for healthy hormones) being dumped into the urine rather than being utilised. Magnesium is needed to produce serotonin.

3 EXERCISE SMARTER NOT HARDER Weight training and low body weight both place stress loads on the body, causing spikes in stress hormones. So short bursts of training will be healthier than slogging it out like a machine. I am a big fan of incidental exercise and activity that uses your whole body, like gardening, spring cleaning or walking instead of driving to the local shops.

4 LOVE YOUR LIVER Second only to gut health is liver health. Your liver is responsible for cleansing the blood and moving out the gunk. It's like a sponge, mopping up the toxins that would otherwise be polluting your body. From a Chinese medicine viewpoint, stress substantially upsets the liver. Consider doing an alkalising cleanse with a short-term, plant-based diet for a week or two, starting each morning with lemon water and ending each day with a probiotic. In just few days you'll begin to feel a million bucks.

5 HEALING THE MIND This is the most powerful tool in the treatment of PCOS. Your thoughts and beliefs influence the way in which your tissues, cells and hormones communicate. We'll learn more about that below.

STRESS

Cortisol and adrenaline increase insulin release

Triggers release cortisol and adrenaline

INSULIN

High insulin levels cause the body to dump magnesium into the urine.

Magnesium is needed to make serotonin.

Upsets serotonin release

Eating sweets leads to increased insulin

Lack of serotonin increases food cravings

How to Manage Endometriosis

Endometriosis is a condition where menstrual blood makes its way into the tissue surrounding the uterus, where it simply shouldn't be. Because of this, it can't readily exit the body. It's literally blood that's stuck or wedged in the body. Through this image, you can imagine how symptoms of endometriosis develop. Stuck objects are painful!

Endometriosis is characterised by:

- painful periods
- clotting menstrual flow
- spotting before the period
- lumps or nodules in the lower abdomen
- bowel troubles (not limited to the period time)
- pain with intercourse
- fertility troubles.

Many women diagnosed with endometriosis are told that pregnancy will be difficult for them. I've found this to be untrue for my clients, as together we can always work out how to treat their condition. Given the right care, healing is absolutely possible.

I find it fascinating that in our modern world there are such large gaps in scientific knowledge.

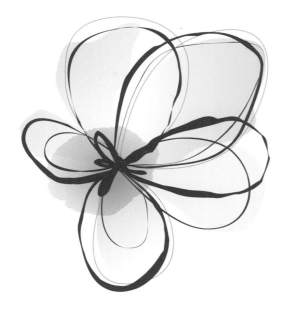

We don't fully know why endometriosis happens. But I know very well the symptoms that my clients experience that help me diagnose it and shape effective treatment. Suspected endometriosis is difficult to confirm without a laparoscopy, but everyone will benefit from making changes to treat the troubling symptoms.

Here's what we know for sure: endometrial tissue travels down through the uterus and out through the cervix. Blood also may travel upward through the fallopian tubes and out into the peritoneal cavity. It's only a small amount of blood that may travel upward but it may carry with it old bits of the endometrial lining. Women who experience extremely painful menstrual cramps are more likely to lose menstrual flow up towards the fallopian tubes. At this point, the blood (and tissue) will either be reabsorbed or may remain and establish itself somewhere within the pelvic cavity—in reality this shouldn't be here. If the body is too weak to reabsorb the blood, stagnation will occur: this is endometriosis.

The endometrial tissues that grow outside the uterus will either be non-pigmented or pigmented (containing blood vessels). Pigmented tissue begins to act like uterine endometrium at period time, which means it reacts to hormones and behaves just like the uterine lining does each month as it prepares to shed—which we experience as monthly bleeding. This type of endometriosis is the most likely to be marked by pain. Non-pigmented types of endometriosis may be associated with fertility trouble for reasons not fully understood.

No matter what your diagnosis is, almost all conditions will benefit from eating to support hormone health. After all, your hormones are the master controllers of your entire body.

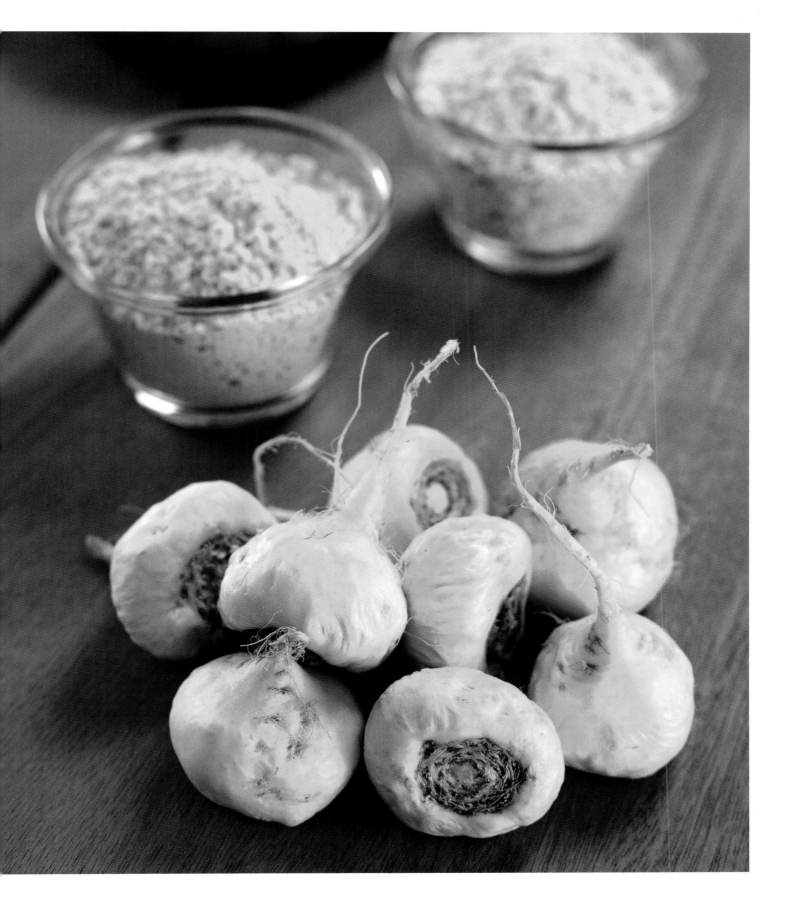

Inflammatory foods place load on the gut and also affect conditions like endometriosis. Become aware of which foods upset the balance—it's like a speed-dial to recovery!

There are things you can do to treat endometriosis that don't involve surgery. But whether you are having surgery or not, it's important to make changes to your diet and lifestyle to keep it from either coming back or getting worse.

Anything inflammatory will worsen endometriosis. Foods that cause inflammation and disrupt gut function include:

- refined foods (like fast food)
- spicy foods
- dairy
- meat (if poorly prepared)
- sugars/fructose.

Cold, raw foods can aggravate and worsen symptoms of endometriosis. I ask my clients to experiment and try four weeks of limiting raw and refrigerated foods. Remember that your body speaks to you through symptoms, so if you find that by doing this your digestion and menstrual symptoms are lessened, continue with it for at least three menstrual cycles to really allow the body to heal.

Just like with PCOS, any stress load on the body will worsen symptoms. This extends to exercise, emotional wellness and general lifestyle. Gentle to moderate exercise is much better for you than high intensity. Physical activity will help to manage endometriosis for many women, as it assists in moving the stuck endometrial blood out of the body.

Finally, feminine hygiene products need to be considered. It's been reported that women who use organic, toxin-free sanitary products noticed improvement in the level of pain and clotting during their periods. Anything that irritates the body will lead to inflammation and pain, so I always recommend organic pads to women with endometriosis. Using tampons may contribute to limiting and hampering blood flow.

There are a few more tips I suggest to those with endometriosis. Consider:

- abdominal massage
- meditation (especially to help with pain management)
- building emotional health
- simple heat packs over the lower abdomen to encourage blood flow.

Many women are able to manage their endometriosis without surgery. Adjusting diet and lifestyle is a must for healing, and the principles and foods to help you do this are all outlined in this book.

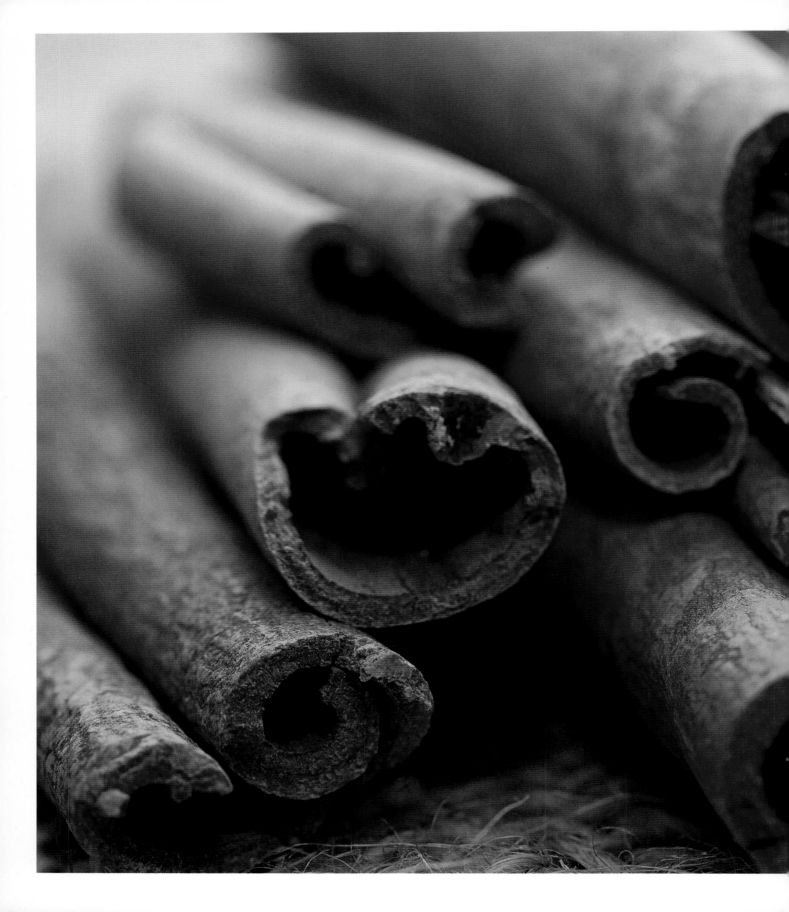

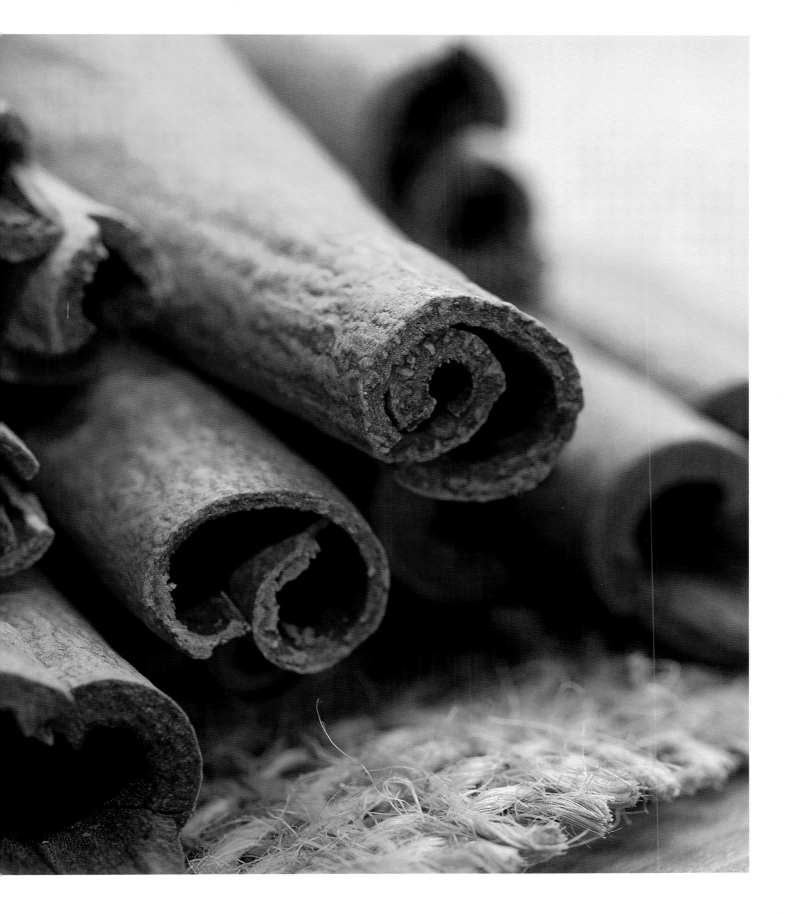

Rebalancing Hormones and Oestrogen Dominance

Oestrogen dominance is currently taking centre stage when it comes to hormone imbalance. It simply means that there is excess oestrogen in relation to progesterone in the body.

Signs of oestrogen dominance include:

- painful, heavy, clotting or long periods
- Mittleschmerz (ovulation pain)
- facial hair—especially above the lip
- PMS, including emotional upset, frustration, anger, headaches, breast distention, nose bleeds, sinus issues, bowel irregularities that occur from ovulation (up to two weeks prior to the period).

Female hormone balance also guides social, sexual and nurturing behaviours. Symptoms of depression, mood swings and anxiety can all stem from oestrogen dominance, and the bubbliest of women may no longer be the life of the party. This happens because progesterone has a specific role in heightening our moods and making us feel happy. It's all about the balance!

Here's the thing that makes many of my clients sit up: Because oestrogen is an anabolic hormone, an excess may lead to weight gain, especially around the abdomen.

As oestrogen levels rise, weight control becomes a really tricky task, as fat cells are also responsible for producing oestrogen. So the more fat cells we have, the more oestrogen

Research has shown that having too much or too little oestrogen signals the body to hold on to extra kilos, especially around the waist, thighs, under the bottom and at the tops of the arms.

is released into the body, the more fat cells grow. And on top of that, increased oestrogen contributes to bloating and fluid retention.

Exercise alone for women who are oestrogen dominant will never be enough, because the excess weight is due to misfiring hormones.

But by rebalancing hormones through the right diet in combination with gentle to moderate daily exercise will set the wheels in motion.

When it occurs it's thought that there are several causative factors linked to oestrogen dominance. These include:

- considerable consumption of hormone-supplemented, non-organic meat
- excess copper (think copper pipes, like those in household hot-water systems)
- phytoestrogens (oestrogen-mimicking chemicals found in plastics, some beauty products, foods, including soy products, and in our environment).

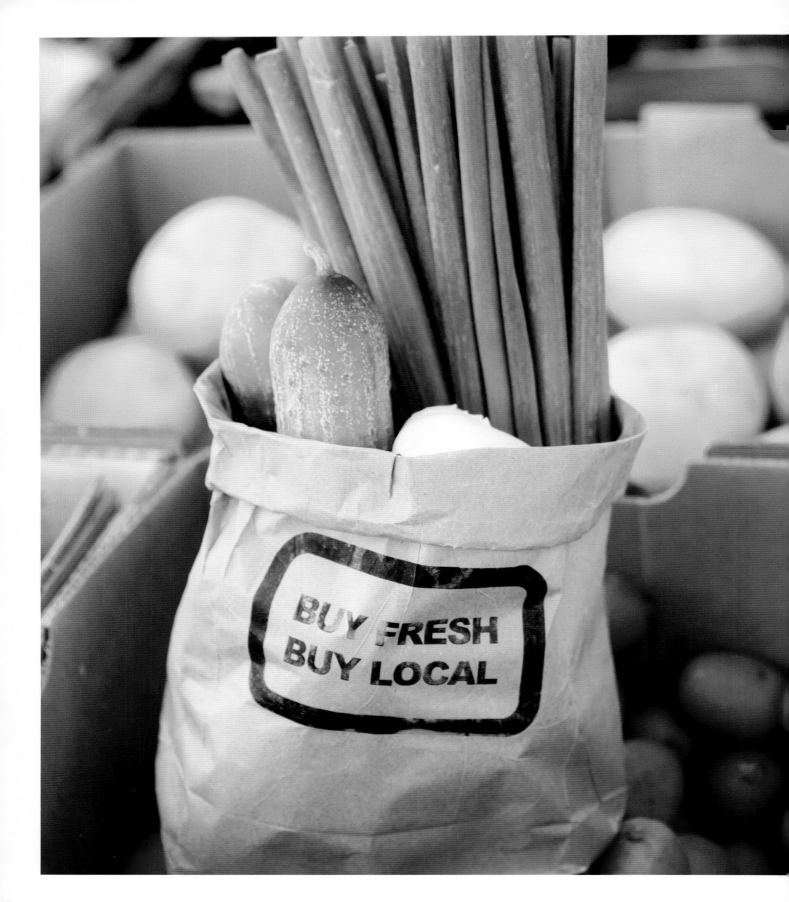

The majority of us have probably consumed hormone-treated meat at some point, drank water out of the hot-water tap or sipped on soy lattes thinking we were reaping the benefits. So if you're scratching your ovaries wondering, could this be me?—don't sweat it. Now you know what to look out for and what to avoid.

Those suffering from polycystic ovarian syndrome, endometriosis, ovarian cysts, breast irregularities and abnormal weight gain very likely have oestrogen dominance to thank. Menopause is also a time where we see oestrogen dominance. This is what causes women to gain weight and feel like they're going a little crazy or out of control. It's a time when we see increased facial hair, especially of the moustache variety. We're forgiven for dreading those transition years, but let me reassure you—menopause doesn't have to be difficult, and if we set ourselves up in our early years, the transition can be a smooth one.

It was once thought that during menopause the ovaries shut down and oestrogen declined. We are now learning that, quite to the contrary, the ovaries play a huge role in menopause and beyond. While their task may change completely, they are equally integral to life after menstruation—so we need to look after them even more carefully in our youth.

Oestrogen dominance is seeing many women suspended in perimenopause. This means that symptoms of menopause act like a worn-out rubber band—they are stretched out for years because the presence of oestrogen is so high. In a healthy system, the adrenal glands take on much of the ovarian function in our post-menstruation years. But if the adrenal

We shouldn't wait until we are older to tackle menopause. Setting up your hormone health begins in your early reproductive years. This truly is the key to long-term overall wellbeing.

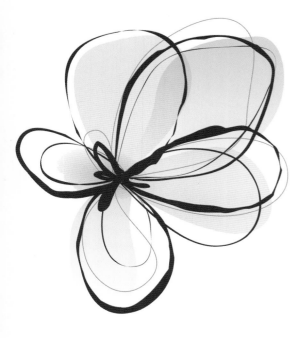

glands are tuckered out, they can't do their job, leading to the lingering state of perimenopause, which is treated with medication much like an illness. As we now know, treating symptoms is not a viable long-term solution. The cause needs to be addressed, so decreasing oestrogen by way of diet and lifestyle is the approach I recommend for treating perimenopause.

For pre-menopausal women with oestrogen dominance, doctors are likely to suggest the pill, simply because there isn't much else on offer. But we all now know that the pill is nothing more than a bandaid solution. Rip off the bandaid and, not only does it hurt, but the condition is still there, and the symptoms often come back ten-fold. Of course, if you're using the pill to control symptoms, when the time comes to make babies you will have your work cut out for you getting back your fertile hormone balance. Let's not forget how the pill affects your body's ability to absorb vitamins and minerals by disrupting your gut flora. And deficient mothers make for deficient babies, a situation that can only compound the effects of postnatal depression, difficult breastfeeding and irritable and colicky infants.

There are some simple changes to your diet that will assist in healing the imbalance, and thereby reduce your symptoms.

Although no one body is the same there are some deficiencies that I see over and over—magnesium is the biggest. It is one of the most important minerals in balancing hormones. Magnesium is a key element in the production of progesterone and is necessary for more than three hundred and fifty different biochemical processes that occur within your body. I recommend that clients suffering oestrogen dominance take a high-dose supplement of magnesium (350 milligrams of elemental magnesium twice daily) for between three and six months.

As a herbalist, I usually prescribe the herb *Vitex agnus-castus* (1 gram per day) alongside magnesium as part of an oestrogen rebalancing program. There are many other herbal formulas that can assist you. I create individual regimens tailored to my clients' specific needs. Consulting a herbalist for an individualised plan will likely get you the quickest results, as it takes into account the other factors in your lifestyle and disposition, as well as your particular symptoms. Self-diagnosis is unlikely to serve you well—always be guided by your health professional if unsure.

As we've discovered, when it comes to happy hormones, a healthy weight range is essential. Remember, a difference of just 4 kilograms can stand between you and your fertility. Improvements in diet and lifestyle will make all the difference.

Taking supplements, along with gentle diet and lifestyle changes and decreasing stress all contribute to balancing oestrogen. Pretty soon those bulges and the mini moustache will be gone, and you'll be looking fabulous (and comfortable) in your jeans!

Remember, the difference of just 4 kilograms can stand between you and your fertility.

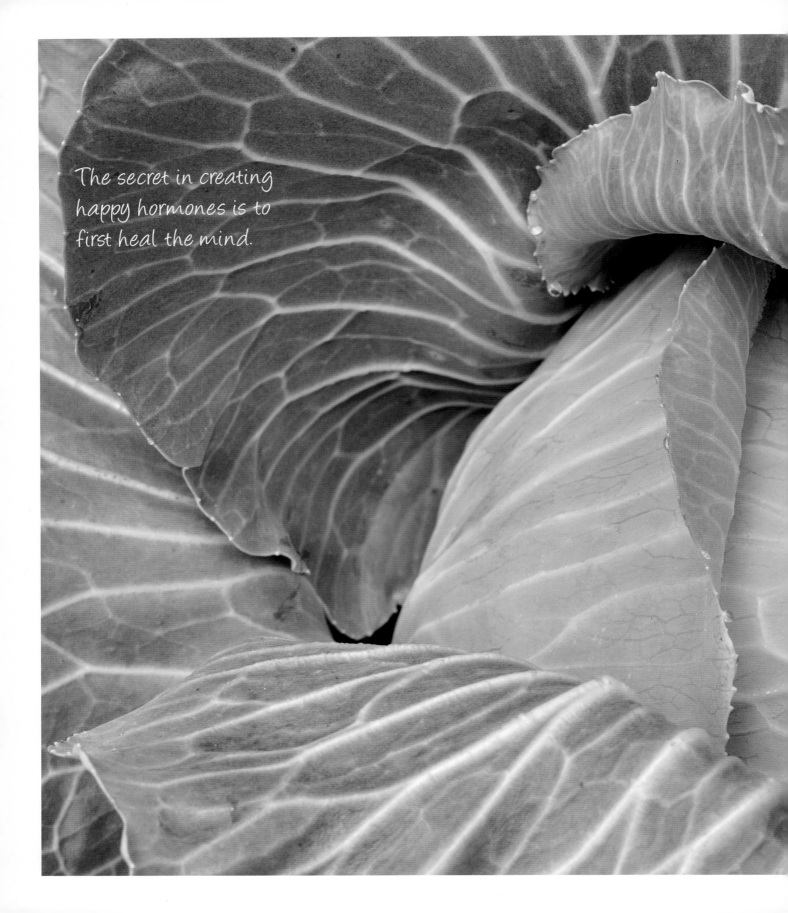

The secret in creating
happy hormones is to
first heal the mind.

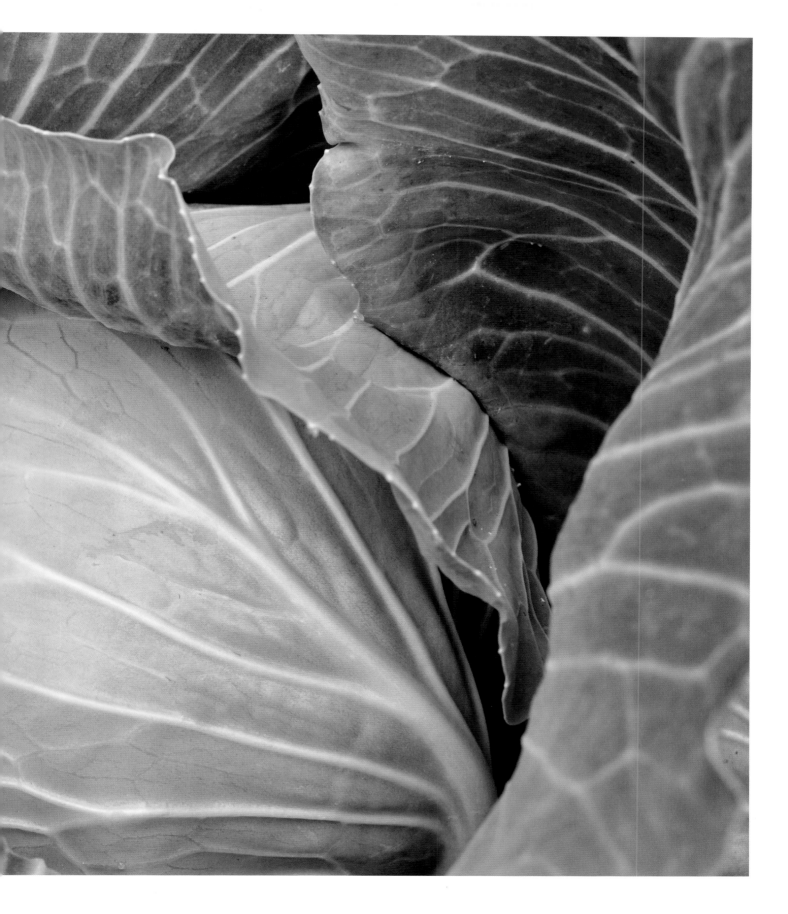

Learning to Love and Healing the Mind

Fertility isn't just about babies. Fertility is much like the earth. Soil that is unnourished, dry and lacking nutrients will rarely grow something beautiful. But if you nurture it, feed it, love it and, most of all, treat it with the respect it deserves, beautiful things will grow and thrive. Your body is just like this. It's capable of amazing blooms. All it takes is care.

When I start talking about fertility, people instantly think of babies or the baby-making years of our life. But fertility is with us for most of our lives, and even post menopause we can keep a sense of fertility. It isn't a hippy or voodoo notion, it is simply a place of all-round nourishment, maintained through all the phases of life.

I recently came across an article by Dr Habib Sadeghi on emotional erosion. It nailed the idea of self-care and self-nurture for women and examined why so many of us are incapable of healing from hormone imbalance. Dr Sadeghi borrowed an idea from John Steinbeck's classic, *The Grapes of Wrath*: when women, the nurturers of humanity, forget how to nurture themselves the consequences are disastrous for our communities, our individual lives, our health, our sense of purpose—everything comes back to self-love and self-care. We simply cannot pass love on to others if we don't love ourselves.

His message was strong. 'When we don't have the proper tools to nurture it, the soil of our soul becomes exposed to the damaging effects of our negative life experiences. It dries up,

Fertility is so much more than conceiving a baby. Fertility is having a thriving reproductive system, much like fertile soil. When the time is right, plant the seed and it will surely grow with the right environment and care.

loses its nourishing capabilities and blows away, leaving us completely ungrounded.' Wow! This was the message I'd been drumming into my clients for so long. We might be all over the physical aspects of our health, but the real health and balance comes from a far deeper place. Dr Sadeghi asks the question: How many people do you know who are flighty, scattered or addicted to drama? We all know those people. They have lost the ability to nourish and nurture their soul through the ups and downs of life. They are missing the tools to get through life's traumas. He went on to speak about how this starts in our childhood—as children our emotional needs aren't always met with compassion. In a perfect world, our parents would comfort us as children, teaching us how to self-regulate our emotions. Instead, we were taught that girls should be pleasers, that it's not okay to show true emotion, and so we learnt to deny our feelings. It is these unresolved traumas that deplete our nutrients. We weren't shown how to apply compassion, empathy and understanding, and we judge ourselves for feeling emotions that we never learnt to express. Repressing emotions is disastrous, as we will only continue to carry the burden around with us—infecting and poisoning our precious soil.

Could our emotional health be the cause of our hormone imbalance? You bet! Unlocking emotional wellness is the only true way to all-round health and wellbeing.

You may not be aware that most of our thoughts are unconscious. Dr Bruce Lipton, the godfather of epigenetics, is at the cutting edge of research into how our thoughts influence the interaction of our cells. He was able to prove that we could influence our genes based on our thoughts and behaviours. Perhaps you know somebody who is always saying, 'I'm sick and tired of this!' I bet they are constantly sick and tired, because that is what they keep reinforcing.

It's a simple fact that we require energy for all our functions as humans.

97% of our thoughts are unconscious—we don't know we are thinking them. But we know that what we think about is what we create. This is called neuroplasticity. Scientists have confirmed that our thoughts, beliefs and environment all shape our wellbeing.

Essentially, we are a big ball of energy being driven by our thoughts and feelings. But if most of your thoughts are unconscious, you may be repeating one or many of the following mantras in your head: I'm not good enough, I'm sick, I'm fat, I'm ugly, I don't have enough money, I'm never going to fall pregnant, I hate my body, I'm sick, I'm tired … You get the picture! These are the messages your body receives all day.

As a mother of a young child with a genetic condition, I see the power of positive thinking and emotional health. My husband and I made a decision when he was diagnosed: we could choose either sickness or wellness. If we chose sickness, we would be consumed by it, but by consciously choosing to foreground wellness, we could focus on that aspect of our child's life. It doesn't mean to say that he won't be unwell at times. In my years as a wellness practitioner it has become

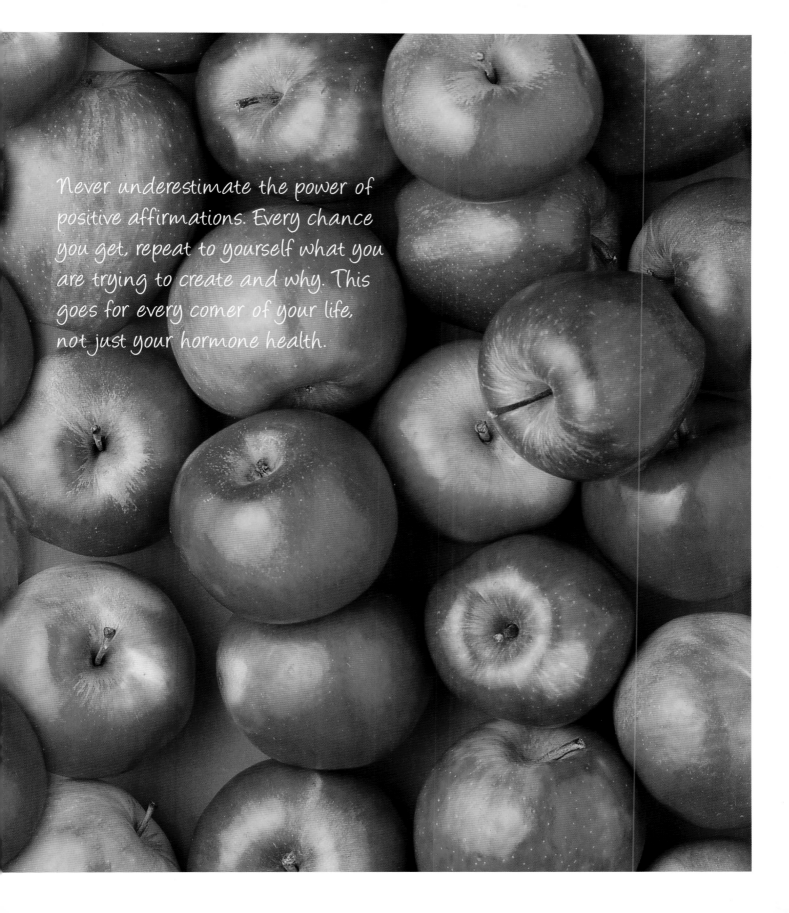

Never underestimate the power of positive affirmations. Every chance you get, repeat to yourself what you are trying to create and why. This goes for every corner of your life, not just your hormone health.

apparent that people who have turned their lives around from serious illness, even cancer, have this mindset, whether its conscious or not. That's not to say that those who have been diagnosed and are afraid wish to be this way, but without the awareness and skill to embrace wellness, it's pretty easy to get caught up in the drama of sickness.

You may not have a serious illness, but even for hormone imbalance or fertility troubles a positive mindset is crucial, because, frankly, that old mantra of yours doesn't seem to be working. Let me guide you through some simple steps towards self-love and emotional wellness. There are also professionals out there who can help you with more in-depth treatment if my tips don't seem to be enough.

First, change the mantra. As your awareness grows, you will be able to catch these unconsciously repeating thoughts. Then, in the moment, you will be able to consciously switch them from negative to positive. The more practice you have catching your negative thoughts, the more awareness and control you will have over your thinking. All of a sudden, you'll find yourself marching to the beat of a different drum—a kinder, more loving, positive rhythm.

If you catch yourself thinking, 'I'm always sick', turn that into, 'I absolutely love being well!' It starts with awareness.

It helps to write down your feelings, be they negative or positive, in a journal. Getting it all out onto paper allows you to understand your thoughts, and what comes out might surprise you! It is from here you can start to create awareness of the thought patterns that aren't serving you.

Practise affirmations. Don't underestimate the power of positive reinforcement. Everybody benefits from praise. Some like a straightforward pat on the back and others might appreciate more subtle forms of acknowledgement. Write yourself sticky notes with affirmations like, 'I love and accept myself completely as I am today, no matter what', or 'my wellness journey serves me each day'. I also like to set myself reminders in my smart phone, so at certain times I will stop, refocus on what I'm trying to create for myself, and then go more lightly through the day. It really is a game changer!

Setting goals and looking ahead is invaluable. If you have a plan, you can always come back to it if you drift off course. This absolutely works for your health and wellness. Set some realistic targets and loosely map out the year ahead. Those who plan, achieve.

Perhaps you've experienced struggles that you've never actually allowed yourself to fully heal from. Enlist the help of a specialist—a life coach or other practitioner who can support you through it. It is so vital that we allow our emotions to be fully felt and experienced in every situation. If you've become good at tucking them away, it's time to examine them, accept them and move on. I can't stress enough how much this will help your wellness and hormone health.

Setting goals and looking ahead is invaluable. If you have a plan, you can always come back to it if you drift off course.

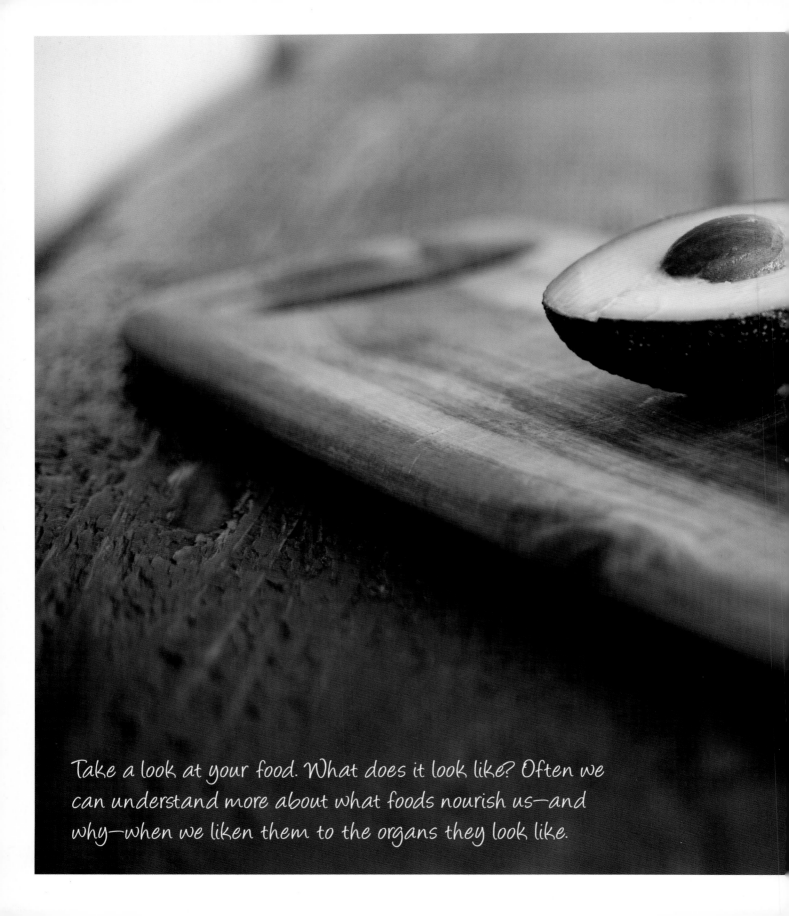

Take a look at your food. What does it look like? Often we can understand more about what foods nourish us—and why—when we liken them to the organs they look like.

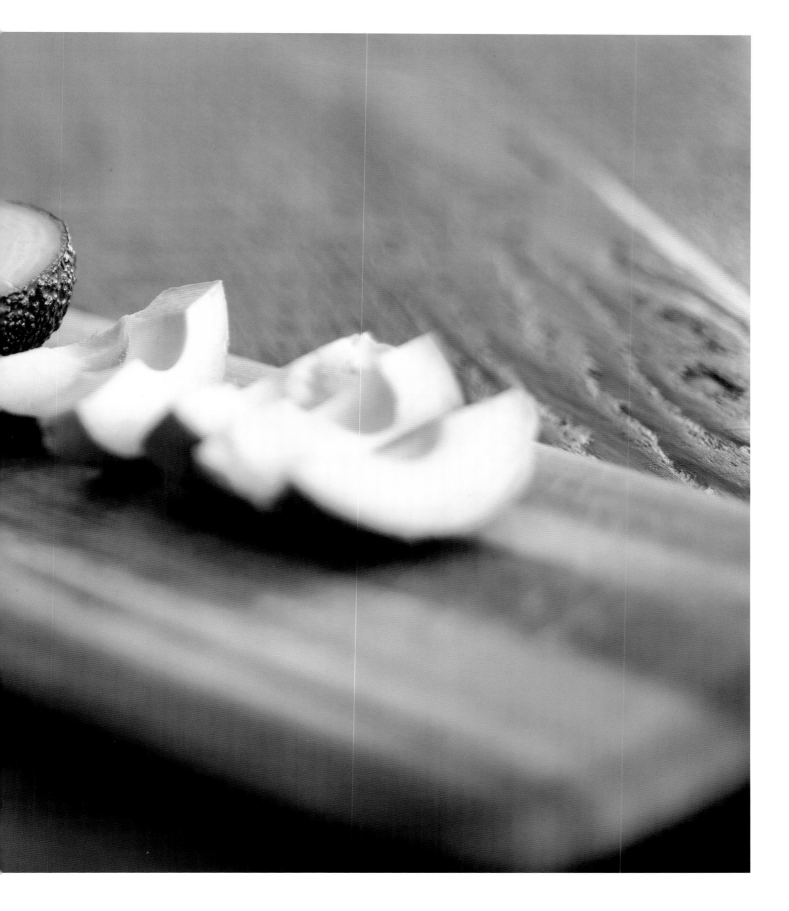

Effortless Weight Loss: Take Control of Your Thyroid

Maintaining a healthy weight relies on hormone balance. As we've learnt, your hormones are the master controllers of all your body's functions.

I see countless women who tell me they have done everything within their power to lose weight, only to continue to see the scales climb. They exercise like Duracell bunnies and get nowhere, or adopt raw vegan diets and keep gaining weight. When my clients need help with weight management, I always ask two questions. Does the food you consume support your unique requirements? And, are your hormones working for you?

Of course, you'll be wondering how you're supposed to know what your unique requirements are. Let your gut be your guide—trial and error is going to be key. If your gut is happy, your hormones will be firing—weight loss and maintenance should become effortless.

Gluten intolerance is often responsible for ongoing gut issues, and it can be completely debilitating to your digestive system, especially your gut lining. As we've learnt, the gut lining is very important in gut health. Gluten is an inflammatory food and, if consumed continually, will create micro tears in the lining, leading food to leak directly into your blood stream. Gluten also triggers an immune response similar to Hashimoto's disease, where the thyroid function is disrupted. It all comes back to the gut and its ability to work well.

Thyroid issues are signs that your hormones need attention. Women with thyroid issues, especially underactive thyroid, have the most trouble with weight maintenance. One of the symptoms of a low functioning thyroid is weight gain, especially around the tops of the legs and arms.

The thyroid is responsible for many hormonal issues—but not all blood tests will capture this.

Here are some signs and symptoms of thyroid dysfunction:
- weight gain around the tops of the legs and arms
- unexplained weight loss (in overactive thyroid)
- tiredness and lethargy
- cold hands and feet
- dry skin
- hair loss
- constipation
- poor memory
- depression.

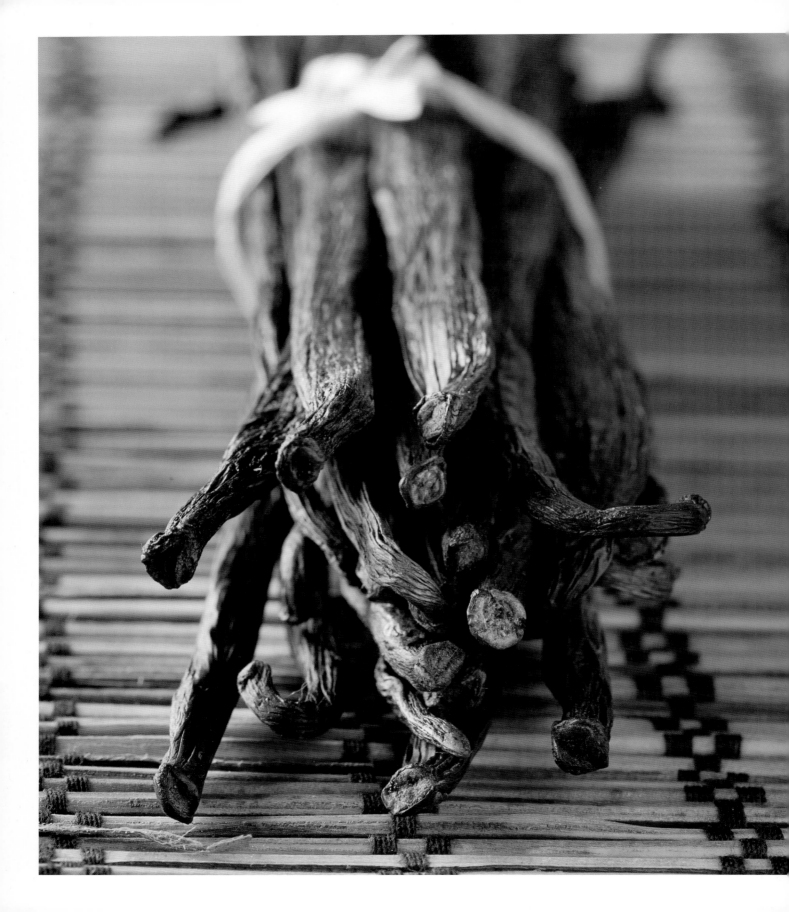

Having one or more of these symptoms is enough to suspect thyroid issues. To treat the cause, you need to rev up your thyroid. There are some simple things you can do to effect this. Increasing progesterone is the main aim. While some practitioners are mad for progesterone creams, I prefer to first suggest diet and lifestyle changes.

Here are my top seven suggestions for progesterone production and thyroid health.

1 MACA It's a superfood from Peru, an adaptogen—so it will respond to your body's unique needs. If your thyroid is underactive, maca helps to fire it up, and if it is overactive it helps slow it down.

2 COCONUT BUTTER OR OIL This boosts your metabolism, is full of good fats that are essential for hormone health and helps the gut work better. Being naturally high in antimicrobial and antibiotic properties, it also assists in healing the gut.

3 SEAWEED High in iodine, seaweeds prop up a slow thyroid. You could alternatively use iodine supplements, but I prefer to use food as medicine. Iodised salt is also a great dietary source. Be mindful that if your thyroid is overactive, supplementing iodine is not recommended.

Always coming back to diet and lifestyle is key. You can sit in your health practitioner's office and have the most amazing treatment, but if you walk out and continue a toxic life, very few changes will occur.

4 SELENIUM, MAGNESIUM AND VITAMIN A
These guys keep your thyroid in check and are
essential for general hormone health. (Keep in mind
that if your gut is compromised, your body may
be having trouble assimilating these nutrients from
your diet.)

5 EXERCISE This is important to stimulate the
thyroid—especially for those who are stressed.
Exercising in short bursts—twenty minutes every
day—is ideal.

6 SLEEP Another vital healer. With exercise, eight
hours of sleep will help to sort out those cortisol
levels and support prolactin.

7 EAT LITTLE AND OFTEN Keeping things chugging
along is a must for those with a sluggish thyroid. They
(I should say 'we', because I'm one of those people!)
require that extra kick to the metabolism.

Of course, sometimes things need a little more tweaking. If
you adopt these changes and feel you're still struggling, your
natural health practitioner is your go-to person.

Connecting the Dots

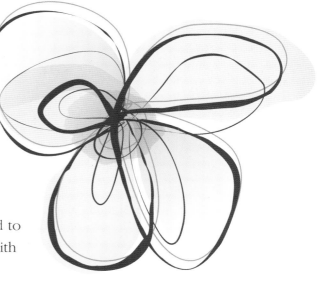

Your gut will start to fire along nicely as you start to incorporate a mix of good fats, proteins and nutrient-rich, high-quality produce, with a little help from probiotics and fermented foods. With this new knowledge you're equipped to navigate the pre-baby and post-baby days and start living with happy hormones.

Remember that symptoms are your body's way of communicating with you—and nothing should interfere with that communication. Medicines like the pill may have set us back, but with newfound awareness you'll be pinpointing ovulation like a professional in no time: whether for contraception or conception, knowing your body as a woman is vital.

Now that you understand the various hormone imbalances, how they can affect weight control and how emotional wellness fits in the mix, you're well on the road to hormone happiness!

'Even if I knew that tomorrow the world would go to pieces, I would still plant my apple tree.'
MARTIN LUTHER

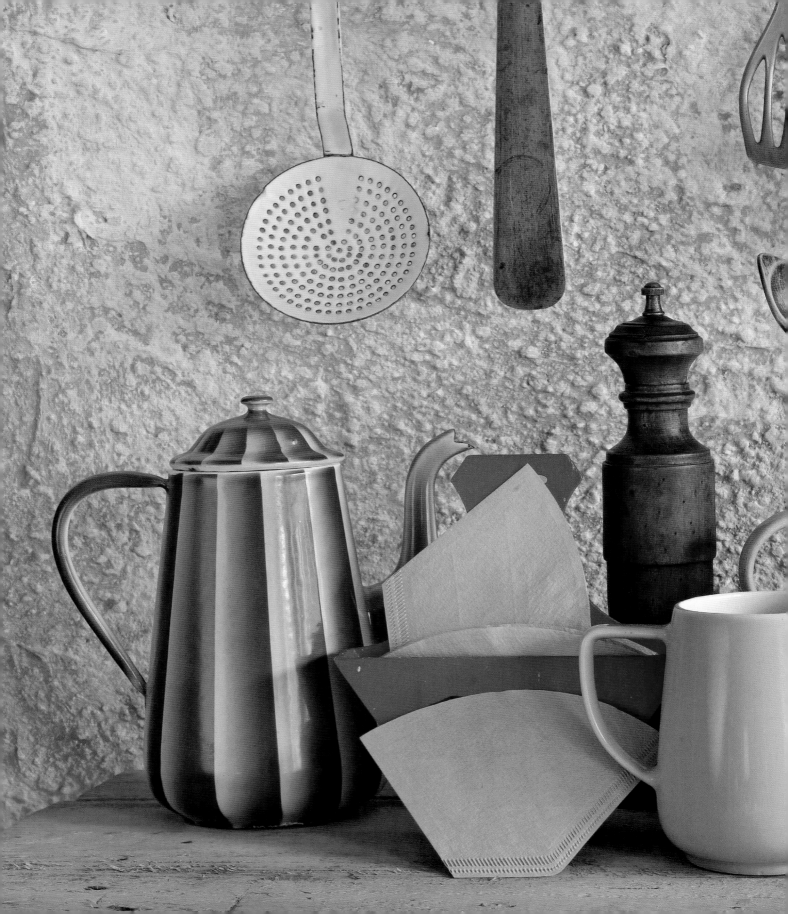

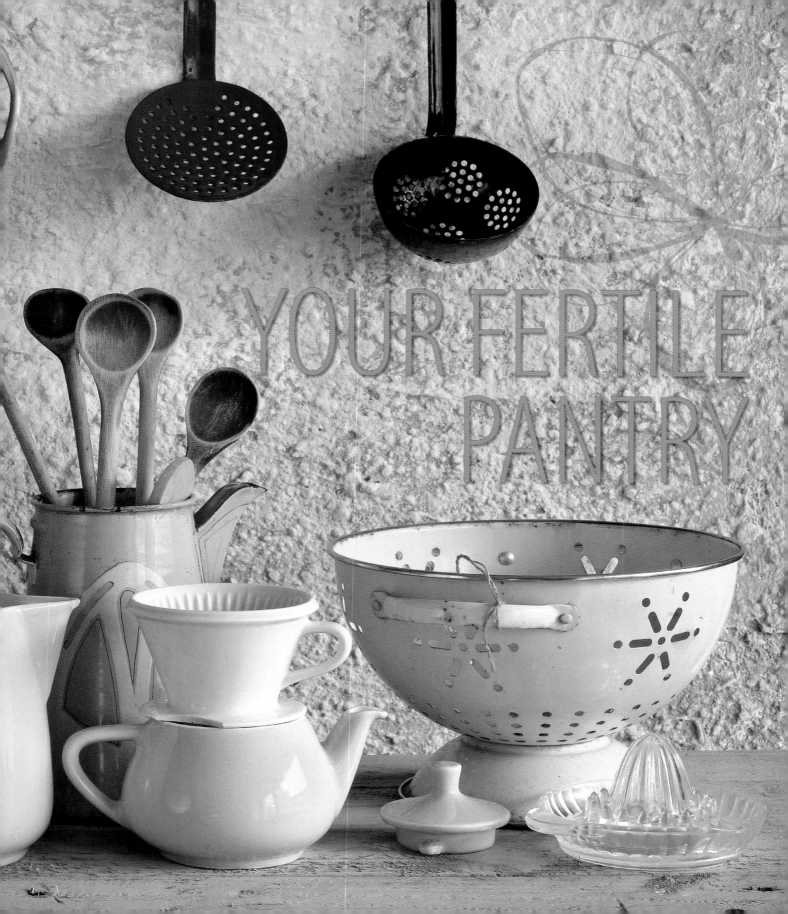

YOUR FERTILE
PANTRY

'Let food be thy medicine
and medicine be thy food.'
SOCRATES

YOUR FERTILE PANTRY

Let's help you get set for a new, fertile way of eating. The easiest
way is to stop buying the bad stuff and fill your pantry
with fertility-promoting fuel foods!

Fertility Must-haves

Avocados, eggplant and pears target the health and function of the womb and cervix—they even look just like these organs. Research shows that when a woman eats one avocado a week, it balances hormones, moves unwanted weight and helps prevent cervical cancers. And, how profound is this—it takes exactly nine months to grow an avocado, from blossom to ripened fruit.

Eating figs increases the motility and quality of men's sperm, assisting in overcoming male sterility. Figs are historically known as an aphrodisiac too—that's a fertility food!

Olives and olive oil assist the health and function of the ovaries.

Eggs! A complete, neatly packaged meal. The perfect balance of fats and protein and a great snack if you're on the run. (I've been known to carry a hard-boiled egg in my handbag!)

Superfoods—think maca, maqui, chia and açaí—great for health and fertility too! Maca is excellent to balance hormones, especially as we get older, and it's great for PMS too.

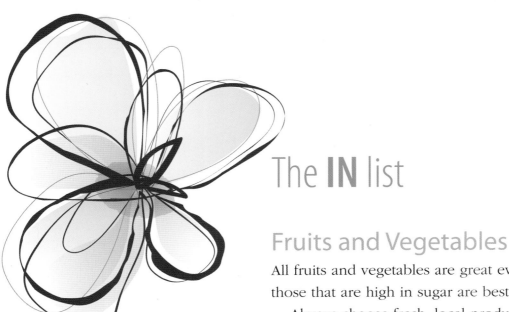

The **IN** list

Fruits and Vegetables

All fruits and vegetables are great everyday foods, although those that are high in sugar are best in moderation.

Always choose fresh, local produce. This approach ensures you are eating what is in season. Read where your produce is grown or flown from. Cherries in the middle of winter? Move on. If you find it difficult shopping for in-season produce there are many delivery services that will do the hard work for you.

Meats and Animal Products

I encourage my clients to choose organic, grass-fed meat and animal products. Grain-fed animals breed abnormal bacteria and are nutritionally lacking, especially in the area of fats (the ratio of saturated fats to omega-3 can be as poor as 20:1, with grass-fed closer to 3:1). Grain-fed animals are bad for our health, which is not surprising—animals are not meant to graze on grains!

Dairy

I personally choose nut milks or goat's milk, but I'm not opposed to cow's milk when we are talking fertility. Opt for organic, non-homogenised milk if you can. The more natural, the better. However, many of us don't tolerate dairy products from cows all that well. The casein protein found in dairy from cows is quite hard on digestion. Goat's milk and goat dairy products are a good alternative. You'll be surprised at just how similar they taste. Rice milk is my other favourite. It doesn't contain hormone-mimicking properties like soy milk does, and it's easy to digest.

Grains, Legumes and Nuts

Soak, soak and soak some more! Why? These guys can be rather hard on the digestive system, and in Australia imported legumes are also chemically treated to make them sterile. Nasty! Soaking removes some of the pesticides and chemicals and helps the gut digest better, lowering the 'gas' factor, and makes cooking easier. By allowing these products to soak, you are setting off the process of fertilisation within what is essentially a seed, which also unlocks the digestive benefits.

To prepare, cover grains and legumes with just enough water and leave to soak overnight. Rinse, and you're ready to rock and roll (as in cook). Keen to activate nuts? See Activated Nuts in Recipes.

Superfoods

Some superfoods are especially good for fertility.
Here are my top five.

1 MACA This is packed with vitamins, minerals, enzymes and amino acids, it balances hormones, is great for PMS, vaginal dryness and depression. It is also said to help regulate menstrual cycles, enhance libido and stimulate fertility! If you only eat one superfood, this has to be it.

2 MESQUITE High in protein as well as vitamins and minerals, it assists in stabilising blood sugar, which is good news for PCOS sufferers and those with thyroid and insulin issues.

3 GUBINGE Local superfood! Bush medicine is very clever.

4 CACAO Chock full of antioxidants, and high in essential minerals to optimise the body's functions, cacao is excellent for fertility!

5 GOJI BERRIES These little gems are like nothing else on the planet! They contain protein and are a great source of trace minerals.

Probiotic Foods

You already know fermented foods and probiotics are great for you because of their gut healing, good-bacteria-promoting properties. Incorporating them into your pantry is the best way of restoring your gut health. These foods can be hard to get, but some of the best can be found in health-food shops, in the forms of sauerkraut and kombucha (fermented tea).

The **OUT** list

Leave the refined, packaged foods on the shelf. One way to think about it is that now you'll do your grocery shopping by only purchasing from the outer aisles of the supermarket, where the fresh food is! There might be a few exceptions, but on your next trip, you'll see what I'm getting at.

Soy Products

Soy gets a pretty bad rap these days, so let's break it down. Organic, non-genetically modified tofu is a great source of protein, which is an important part of your fertility diet. But soy products have their downside. They're heavily processed, which is never good. They also contains phytoestrogens, which as we know can mess with the hormone balance and reproductive workings of the body, especially for men. Non-fermented soy products are difficult to digest, contributing to poor gut health. However, fermented soy products, like miso and tempeh, are easier on the gut. Consume in moderation.

Soy is everywhere—in bread and many refined foods. To avoid eating potentially harmful genetically modified, non-organic soy, get busy in your kitchen and prepare your own foods. That way you know exactly what you are getting.

Gluten

Gluten interferes with everybody's digestion—not just those diagnosed with coeliac disease or gluten intolerance. Why? Because it's hard to digest and causes inflammation in the gut, which compromises your all-round health. As you already know, my advice is to avoid it all together. This especially means all wheat products are off the list. Look for gluten-free pastas, or supplement your diet with brown rice, and other whole grains and seeds, such as quinoa and millet.

Sugar

Our bodies just aren't designed to cope with the amounts of sugar the average person consumes. It is making us sick and tired and, worst of all—fat. And as we know, excess weight affects fertility. It disrupts ovulation and changes the natural balance of hormones. This goes for men too, who have their part to play in fertility. So get the sugar out of the pantry! Try out the natural and safe alternatives like stevia, xylitol and rice malt syrup. They will be kinder to your insides and your waistline.

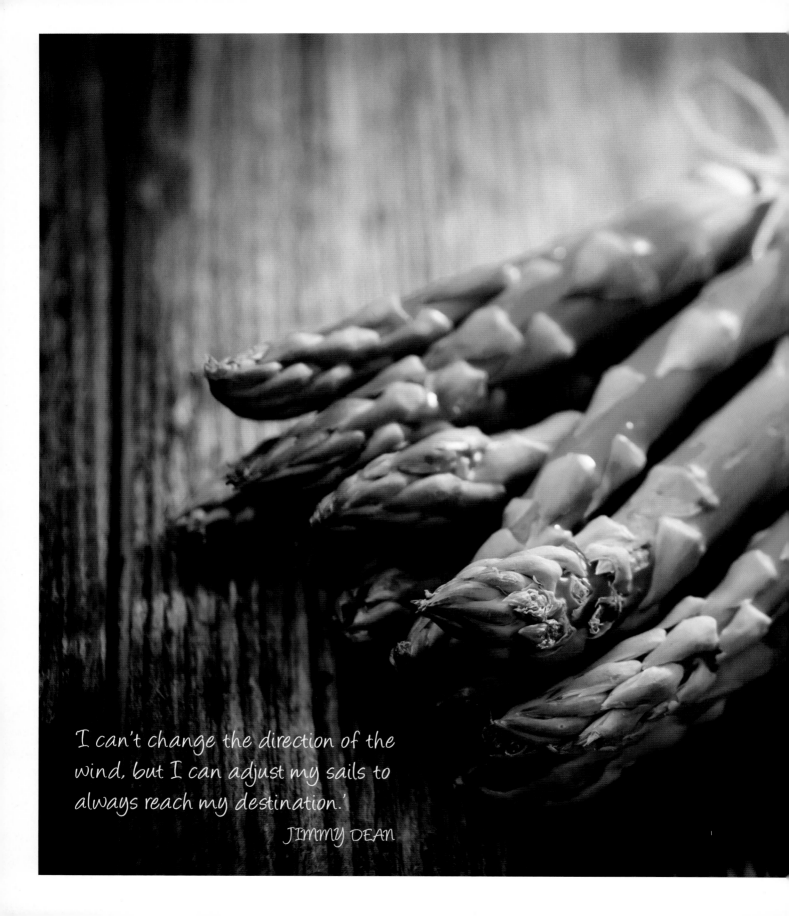

'I can't change the direction of the wind, but I can adjust my sails to always reach my destination.'

JIMMY DEAN

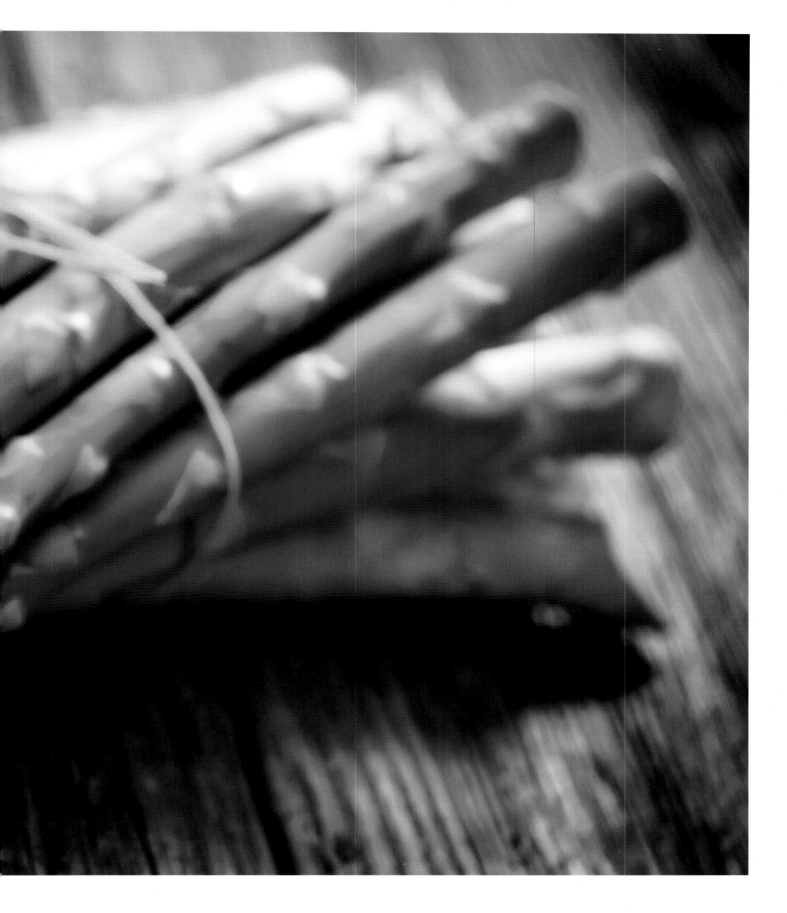

Your Fertile Shopping List

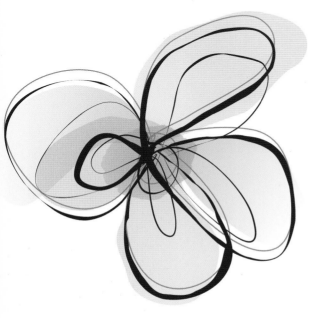

Veggies

asparagus
artichokes
avocado
beans
broccoli
broccolini
Brussels sprouts
cabbage
capsicum
carrot
cauliflower
celery
corn
cucumber
eggplant
endive
garlic
kale
leek
lettuce
mushrooms
onion
parsnips
peas
potato
pumpkin

radish
silverbeet
spinach
sweet potato
zucchini

Fruit

apples
avocado
berries
cherries
citrus (lemons, limes,
    oranges)
currants
dates
figs
mango
pineapple
rhubarb
sultanas
tomato

Grains

brown rice
oats, whole or rolled
quinoa

Legumes

beans
chickpeas
lentils
tapioca

Flour

buckwheat
coconut
millet
rice
spelt

Nuts

almonds
cashews
coconut
hazelnuts
macadamia
walnuts

Dairy and Milks

butter
coconut yoghurt
feta

goat's cheese
goat's milk
haloumi
Parmesan cheese
rice milk
ricotta
yoghurt

Condiments

apple cider vinegar
baking powder
cacao nibs
baking soda
cacao, raw
chilli powder
cinnamon
cocoa
coconut flakes
coconut oil
currants
goji berries
kefir grains
nutmeg
olive oil
vanilla beans
white mulberries

Sweeteners

maple syrup
raw honey
stevia
xylitol

Herbs

basil
coriander
parsley
thyme

And the Rest

apple juice, organic
brown rice protein powder
chicken bones
chocolate, dark
coconut milk/water
corn chips
eggs, organic and
    free range
gubinge
kefir 'grains'
maca powder
maquise
peanut butter

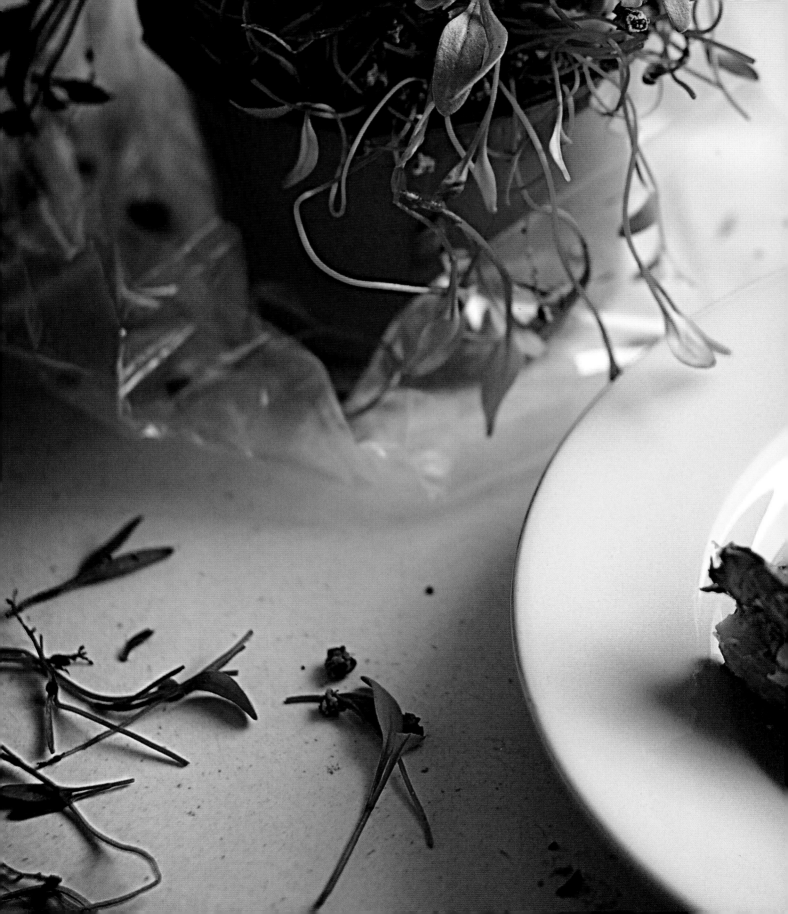

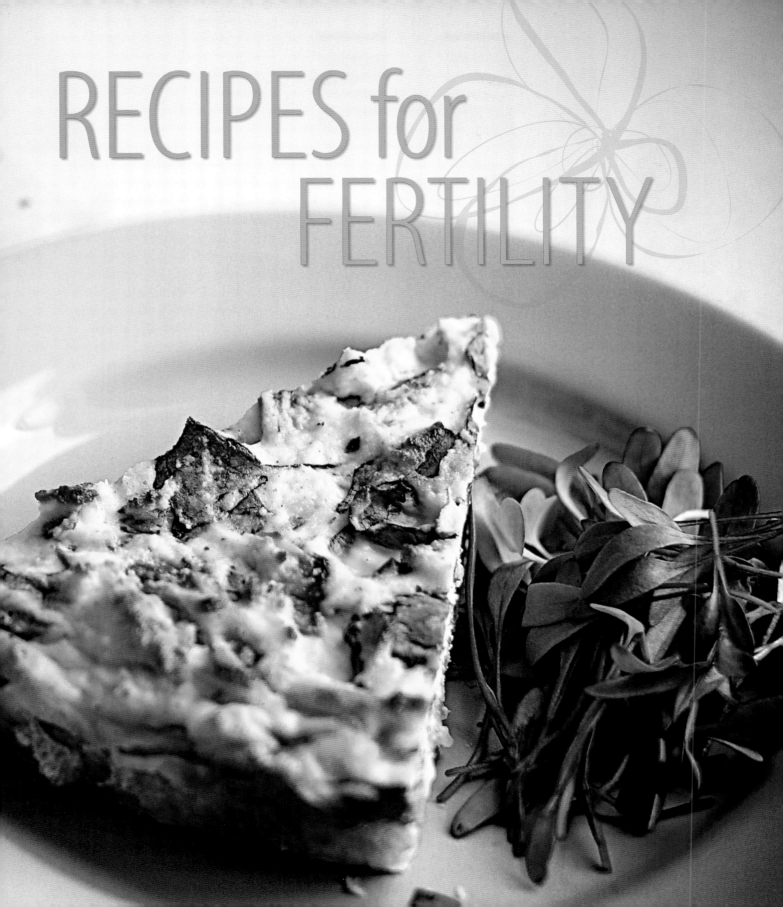

RECIPES for FERTILITY

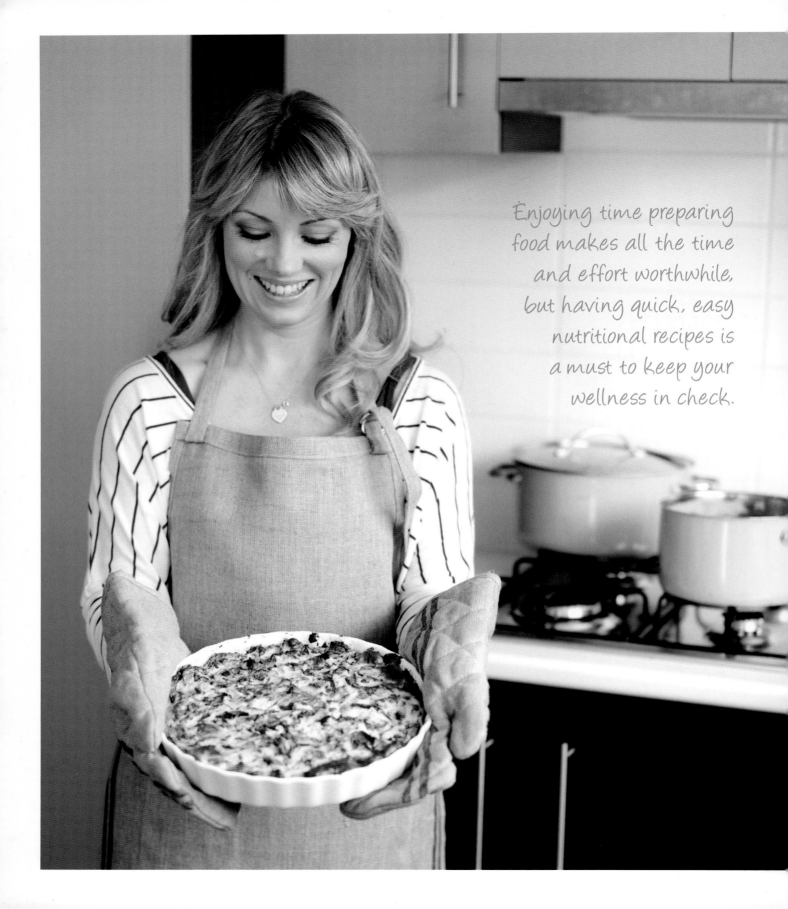

Enjoying time preparing food makes all the time and effort worthwhile, but having quick, easy nutritional recipes is a must to keep your wellness in check.

RECIPES for FERTILITY

Although most of my recipes are vegetarian, animal proteins are a fabulous source of nutrients and should not be ignored for a more fertile you. I've focused on vegetarian recipes to cater for all lifestyles, but if you're a meat eater, you'll easily be able to add the animal protein of your choice, like a piece of steak or a chicken fillet, to these lunch or dinner recipes.

Aim for roughly 90–110 grams of protein per day. Confused about what that looks like? The table below allows you to visualise it. Easy, isn't it?

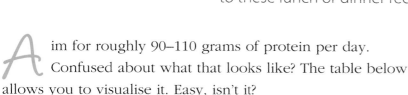

Protein Sample Menu

BREAKFAST	MORNING TEA	LUNCH	AFTERNOON TEA	DINNER
Eggs (20g each)	Apple and peanut butter (10g)	Stir fry with meat or tofu (30g)	Yoghurt and handful of nuts (10g)	Fish and veggies (20g)

Not Too Hot, Not Too Cold

Eat foods that are room temperature or warmer, especially during winter. This supports healthy gut function. Cold foods, on the other hand, lead to phlegm production and other health problems. Women experiencing period pain should especially stay away from cold foods—warm foods will keep the blood circulating. Your gut is happiest when food is at 37°C or thereabouts.

BREAKFAST

Breakfast sets the tone for your day, and eating protein in the morning is the best thing you can do in the quest for fertility.

When you start the day with sugary cereals on the other hand, your blood-sugar levels peak and then crash shortly afterwards, as does your energy. Then you'll start craving sugar again mid morning and probably succumb to grabbing a muffin or muesli bar (full of sugar). And so the cycle can continue all day, with your sugar levels yo-yoing up and down. But if we get a protein fix in the morning we won't get these same peaks and dips. We are satisfied for longer, our minds are sharper and we don't get distracted by cravings. Also great news for your gut and, naturally, for your fertility.

Granola

MAKES 10 SERVINGS

You will need two baking trays.

5 cups whole oats (or a rolled grain mix)
3 cups walnuts, roughly chopped
1 cup mixed nuts, roughly chopped
½ cup sunflower seeds
½ cup almond meal
1 cup mashed, stewed apple (see Stewed Fruits)
1 cup liquid from the stewing process
3 tbsp coconut oil, melted

❶ Preheat oven to 180°C. Add the wet to the dry ingredients and mix well, adding more stewing liquid if the dries are not evenly coated.

❷ Line two trays with baking paper and divide mixture evenly between the two. Bake for 40–50 minutes, turning mixture with a fork every 10 minutes until it is quite dry and completely golden.

❸ Allow to cool and store in an air-tight container in your pantry for up to a month. You can also add any kind of dried fruit. I like chopped dates and currants. Enjoy with your preferred milk as a breakfast or dessert.

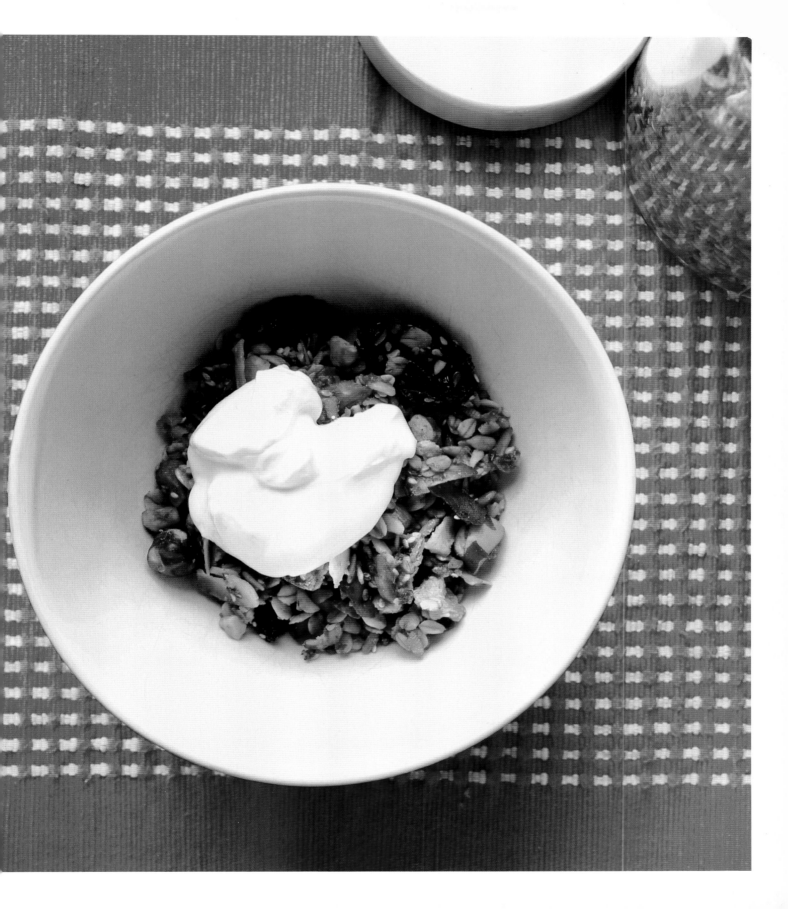

Beginner's Green Smoothie

MAKES 1 LARGE SMOOTHIE

You will need a handheld or bench-top blender.

1 big handful baby spinach
  (or preferred greens)
1 lemon, peeled and roughly
  chopped
1 cucumber, peeled and roughly
  chopped
1–2 sticks celery, roughly
  chopped
1 frozen banana
1 tbsp coconut oil
300ml coconut water (or water)
4–6 ice cubes (optional)

❶ Blend all ingredients for
  30 seconds, serve and enjoy!
  If it's too thick add a little more
  water. Great for first thing in
  the morning but also for lunch,
  dinner or a snack.

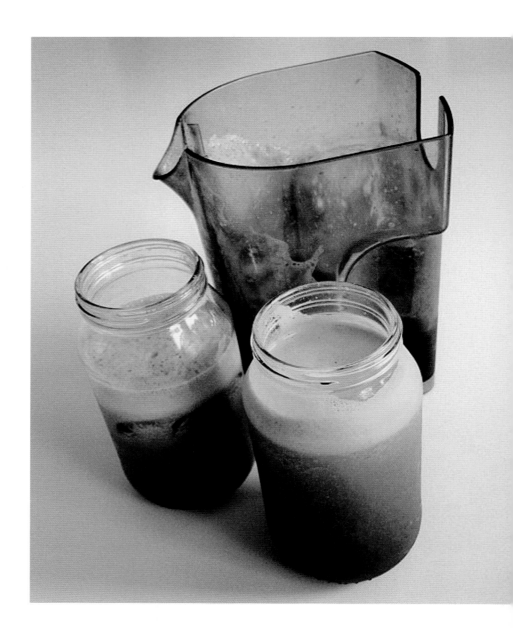

Poached Eggs
with Tomato Salad

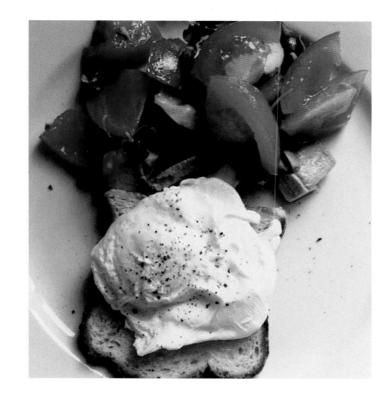

SERVES 1

You will need a medium saucepan.

1.5L water

2 tbsp apple cider vinegar

2 eggs, room temperature

2 tomatoes, diced

1 avocado, diced

handful basil leaves

olive oil

salt and pepper

❶ Bring water to boil in your saucepan and add vinegar to assist the poaching process. Stir boiling water to create a small whirlpool in the centre and crack in an egg at a time, cooking each one separately.

❷ Cook for 2–3 minutes for a soft yolk and 3–4 for a set yolk.

❸ To prepare the tomato salad, combine the tomatoes and avocado with torn basil leaves. Drizzle with olive oil and a dash of vinegar and season with salt and pepper before tossing.

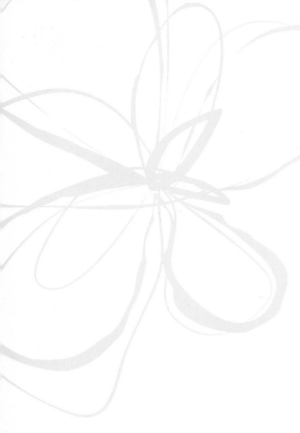

Kefir Yoghurt

You can use raw milk, nut milk (like almond or cashew) or coconut milk. You'll need to search online or ask at your local health food shop for the kefir 'grains'—these are a living culture full of good bacteria. Keeps for three days in the fridge.

MAKES 1 CUP YOGHURT

kefir grains
1 cup preferred milk

❶ Add the kefir grains to the milk. Cover the container and allow the mixture to ferment on your kitchen bench overnight, or up to 24 hours. Note that the longer you leave it, the sourer it will become.

❷ To stall the bacteria, pour the yoghurt through a strainer to remove the grains and place them in a fresh cup of milk in the fridge until you are ready to repeat the process. The grains can be reused indefinitely.

❸ Have this yoghurt in your smoothies, over your granola or eaten like a spoonful of medicine. It's an easy way to get your daily probiotic dose.

Aim to make breakfast the largest meal of the day so your body doesn't have to work overtime digesting a huge meal while you sleep.

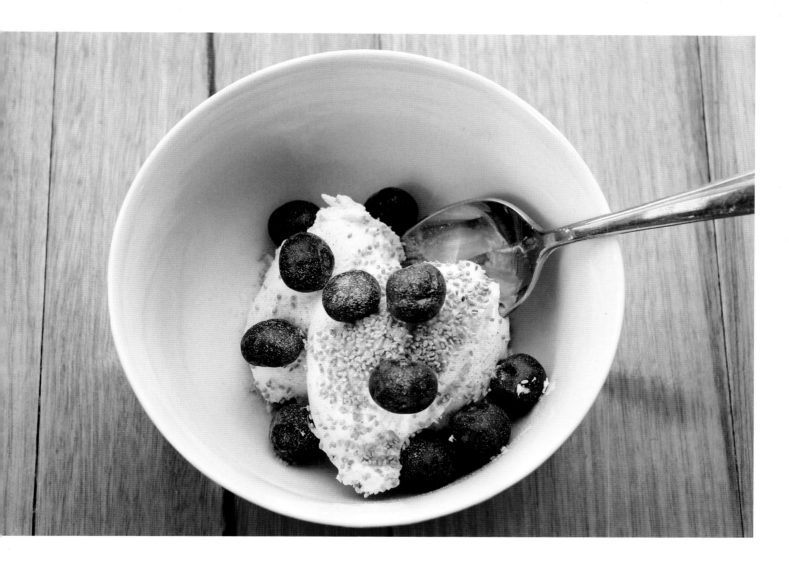

Yoghurt and Berries

Simply combine your favourite berries with your preferred choice of yoghurt.

❶ Don't forget to sprinkle with your favourite toppings—anything from seeds and nuts to other assorted superfoods, such as maca, mesquite or macqui, along with more nutritious additions like cacao and chia seeds.

❷ You can easily make as little or as much as you require, adjusting the servings to your needs—the world is your oyster with this beauty.

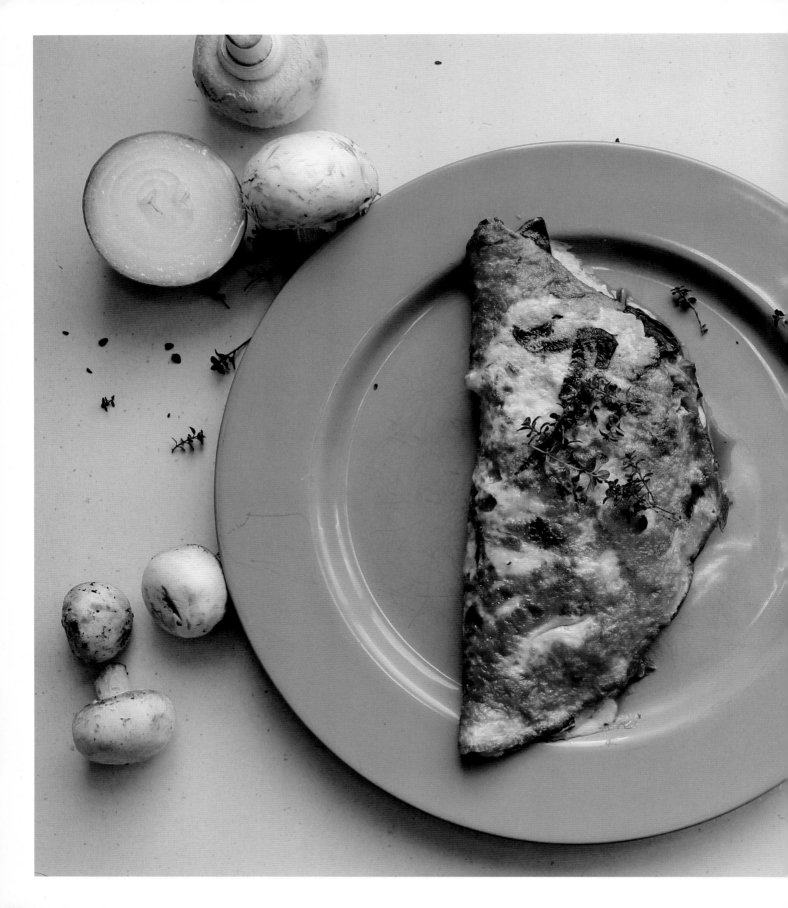

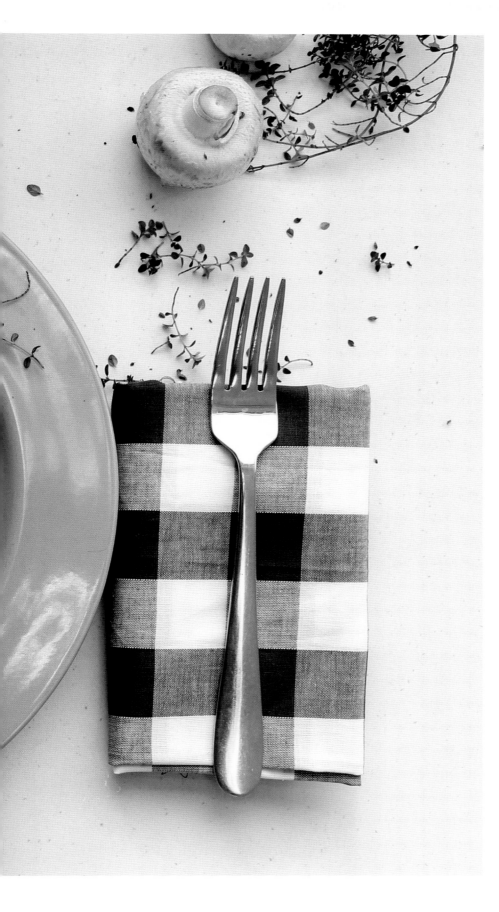

Omelette

SERVES 1

You will need a medium-sized fry pan.

2 eggs
3–4 mushrooms, thinly sliced
½ red onion, thinly sliced
handful spinach leaves
½ tomato, diced
1 tbsp olive oil

❶ Whisk eggs together and then add in mushrooms, onion, spinach and tomato and combine.

❷ Heat the oil in your pan over a medium heat and add the egg mixture. After around 2 minutes, when the egg is almost cooked through, flip with a spatula and cook for a further 30 seconds.

❸ Turn out, and serve.

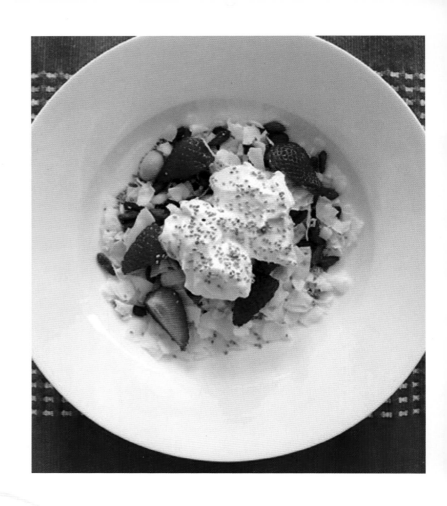

Fertile Muesli

I recommend topping the muesli with yoghurt (my favourite is coconut yoghurt, available at all good grocers) and fresh berries.

MAKES 2–4 SERVES

1 cup of coconut flakes

¼ cup chia seeds

½ cup macadamia nuts

¼ cup cacao nibs

¼ cup goji berries

¼ cup white mulberries

yoghurt and fresh berries for topping

mint to garnish (optional)

1 Simply combine all the ingredients in a bowl.

Samantha Gowing's Morning Smoothie

MAKES 1 LARGE SMOOTHIE

**You will need a handheld or
bench-top blender.**

1 tbsp vanilla protein powder

1 tbsp raw cacao

1 tbsp maca powder

1 cup frozen berries

2 cups your preferred milk or
 coconut water

❶ Blend all ingredients until
 smooth, transfer to a glass and
 enjoy. A meal for any time of
 the day and an easy way to
 have a serve of protein if you're
 in a rush.

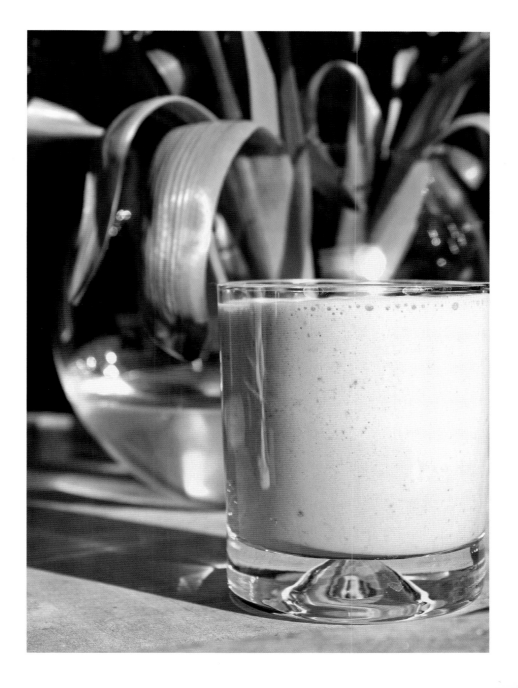

Stewed Fruit

Fruit is easy to stew, and most firm fruits stew well. Simply remove the peel or rind, chop roughly, add just enough water to cover and simmer on the stove until soft. Use a combination of fruits to spice things up, like rhubarb with pear—sweet and sour flavours combine well. You can even stew prunes for a delectable treat—sprinkle with granola and yoghurt for a treat worth sharing!

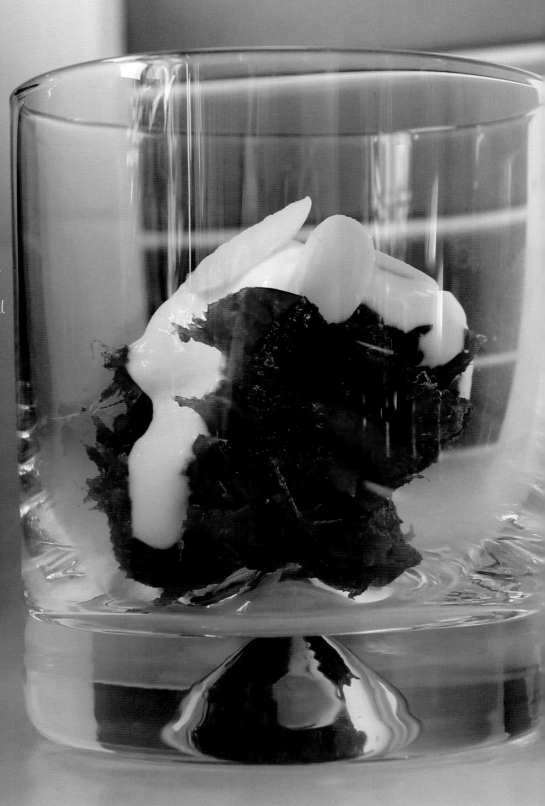

Choosing Your Yoghurt

The type of yoghurt you eat is important. Natural, non-sweetened yoghurt is the bomb, it even aids weight loss. Organic is always best, but if your grocer doesn't stock organic, you can't go past natural Greek yoghurt.

Need it a bit sweeter? You're better off adding a smidge of honey than buying something that is already sweetened—that way you know exactly what you're getting.

Remember what we know about whole foods. Steer clear of low-fat versions. They're often full of extra sugars and you will need more of it to be satisfied, as a fat promotes the feeling of fullness.

Let's not forget that yoghurt is packed full of great bacteria and will certainly support digestion. It's a food that can be eaten every day—as an accompaniment for savoury or sweet foods, or just on its own.

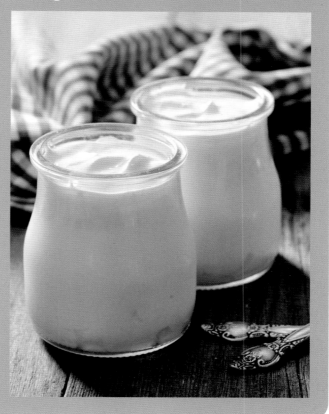

SNACKS

Snacks play a big part in your fertile diet. They'll help you keep up your protein levels, and stop you craving sugars. Not everybody needs to eat snacks, but if you find yourself falling asleep at your desk around 4pm, grab one of these instead of racing to the vending machine.

Activated Nuts

This recipe calls for almonds, but you can use any kind of nuts. You will need to keep your oven on for 12 hours on a low heat, and you will need a glass jar in which to store the nuts.

1 pack raw almonds

❶ Soak the almonds in water overnight.

❷ In the morning, preheat your oven to 60°C. Drain almonds and place on a baking tray. Heat in the oven for at least 12 hours. Cool, and store in a glass jar in your pantry.

❸ Munch on these for a 4pm pick-me-up, or anytime you like.

Activated Goodness

If you decide to try only one recipe from this book—this is it. Activated Nuts. Why? Well, when you soak nuts, they begin to sprout—activating all the goodness. By eating these as a snack, you're doing your digestive system a big favour.

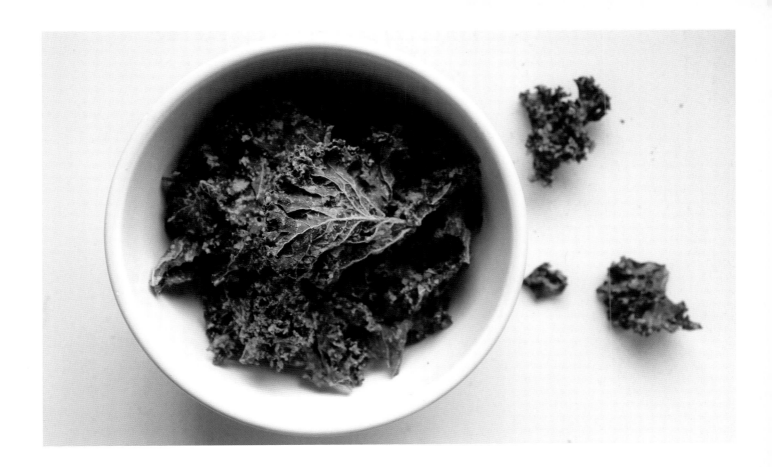

Baked Kale Chips

MAKES A SMALL BATCH FOR 1 OR 2 PEOPLE
You will need a baking dish or tray.

several large kale leaves
2–3 tbsp olive oil
generous pinch sea salt

❶ Preheat oven to 180°C. Tear the leaves by hand into smallish pieces (roughly potato-chip size), being sure to pull away the stem of the leaf (it becomes tough when baked). In a bowl, place kale and oil and toss to cover evenly. Sprinkle salt over kale and toss again.

❷ Line your baking dish or tray and scatter the kale over it.

❸ Bake for approximately 10 minutes, then turn down the heat of the oven to 100°C. Bake until the chips begin to shrivel and are crispy (roughly another 10 minutes).

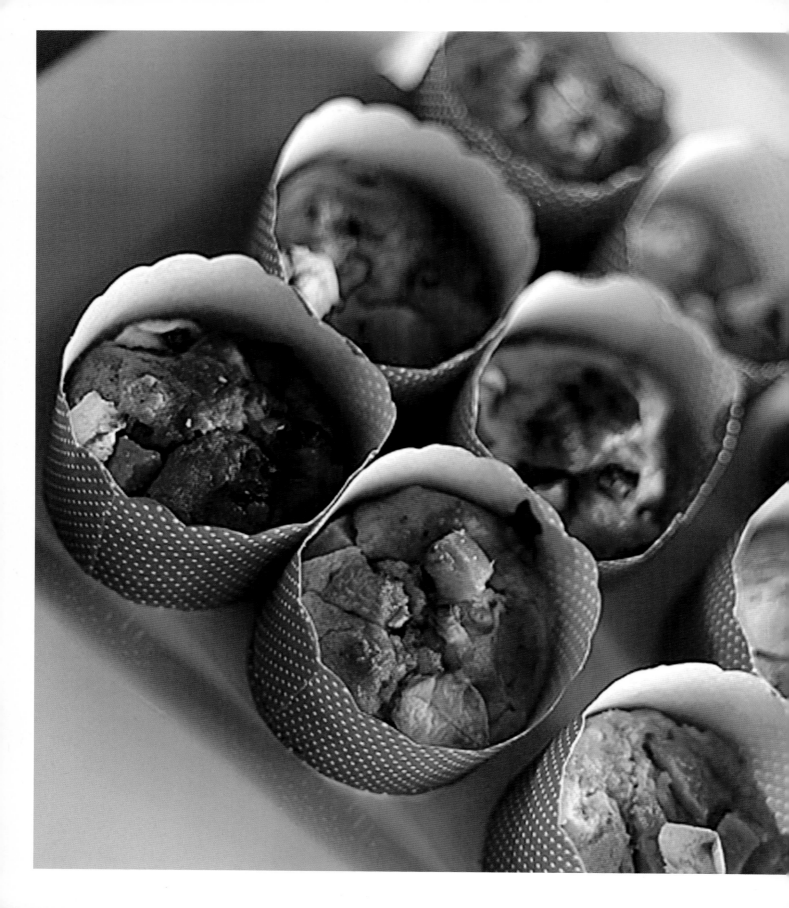

Feta and Pumpkin Muffins

MAKES APPROXIMATELY 12

You will need a muffin tin and a whisk.

2 cups pumpkin, in 1–2cm cubes

2 tbsp olive oil

salt and pepper to season

200g feta

100g Parmesan cheese

leaves of 4–5 sprigs of thyme

2 tbsp seeded mustard

black pepper

3 tbsp pine nuts

1 cup your preferred milk

2 eggs

1½ cups of spelt flour

½ cup of millet flour

3 tsp baking powder

1. Preheat oven to 180°C. Place pumpkin in a baking dish. Drizzle with olive oil and season with salt and pepper. Bake for 20 minutes or until cooked through. Keep oven on.

2. Meanwhile, grease tins—enough for 12 muffins.

3. Once pumpkin has cooled slightly, combine ¾ of the pumpkin, ¾ of the feta, Parmesan, thyme, mustard, pepper and pine nuts and mix briefly to combine.

4. In a separate bowl, combine milk and eggs with a whisk. Add to the pumpkin mixture and fold through briefly with a wooden spoon—taking care that the pumpkin and feta remain intact. Sift in flours and baking soda and again mix briefly to combine.

5. Scoop mixture into muffin tins, filling each case to no more than halfway. Decorate each muffin with remaining pumpkin and feta. Bake for approximately 20–25 minutes, or until the tops become hard and golden.

Buckwheat Muffins with Carrot and Macadamia

If you're avoiding fruit sugar, you can substitute the apple and dates for stevia powder, or even with 1 cup of pureed pumpkin.

MAKES 6–8

You will need a muffin tin (the number of muffins will depend on the capacity of the cases in your muffin tin)

100g buckwheat flour

1 tsp cinnamon

1 tsp salt

1 tsp baking powder

1 tsp baking soda

1 carrot, grated

½ cup stewed apple

½ cup of stewed dates

seeds of 1 vanilla bean

½ cup coconut butter melted

2 eggs, lightly beaten

¼ cup your preferred milk
  (I used goat's milk)

½ cup chopped macadamia nuts

goat's cheese to serve (optional)

1. Preheat oven to 180°C. Grease your muffin tin.

2. In a bowl, combine flour, cinnamon, salt, baking powder and baking soda. Mix well with a wooden spoon.

3. In a separate bowl combine carrot, apple, dates (or pumpkin or stevia), vanilla seeds, coconut butter, eggs and milk, and mix well.

4. Add the wet ingredients to the dry ingredients, partially mixing before adding the macadamia nuts. Mix once more, briefly, until just combined.

5. Spoon mixture into your muffin tin, filling each case no more than half. Bake for 20–30 minutes—until a skewer comes out clean.

6. Once cool, serve with a dollop of goat's cheese on top! Delish!

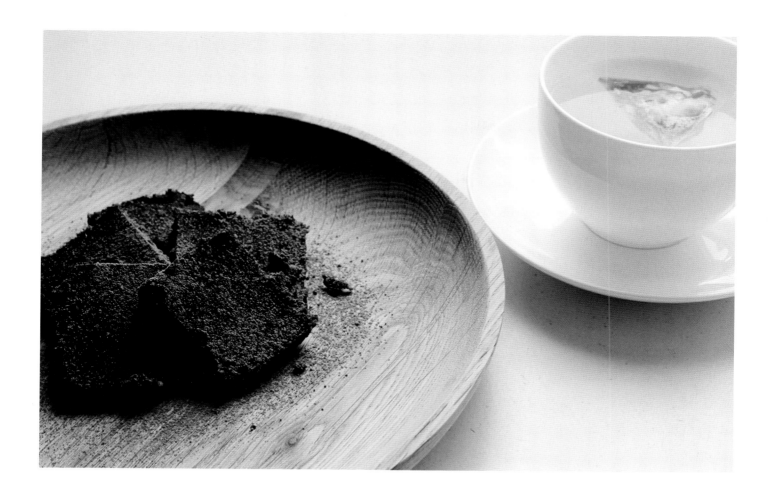

Raw Brownies

MAKES 1 TRAY

You will need a food processor and a brownie tray or slice tin.

3 cups walnuts

1 cup raw cacao

¼ tsp salt

2 cups medjool dates,
  pips removed

❶ In a food processor, pulse walnuts until roughly chopped. Add the cacao and salt and pulse several times to combine. Add the dates one at a time, and keep pulsing until the mixture resembles breadcrumbs.

❷ Line your tray or tin with baking paper and pack mixture firmly inside, pressing down until it resembles a slice. Set in fridge for a minimum of 20 minutes.

❸ Cut into small squares and sprinkle with cacao to serve.

Homemade Pesto

MAKES 1–2 CUPS

Keeps up to 4 days in the fridge.

You will need a food processor.

½ bunch of broccolini

2 cups of basil

3 cloves garlic

1 cup of cashews

⅓ cup olive oil

juice of one lemon

1 tsp salt

❶ Combine all ingredients together in a food processor until smooth.

❷ Serve with your favourite crackers.

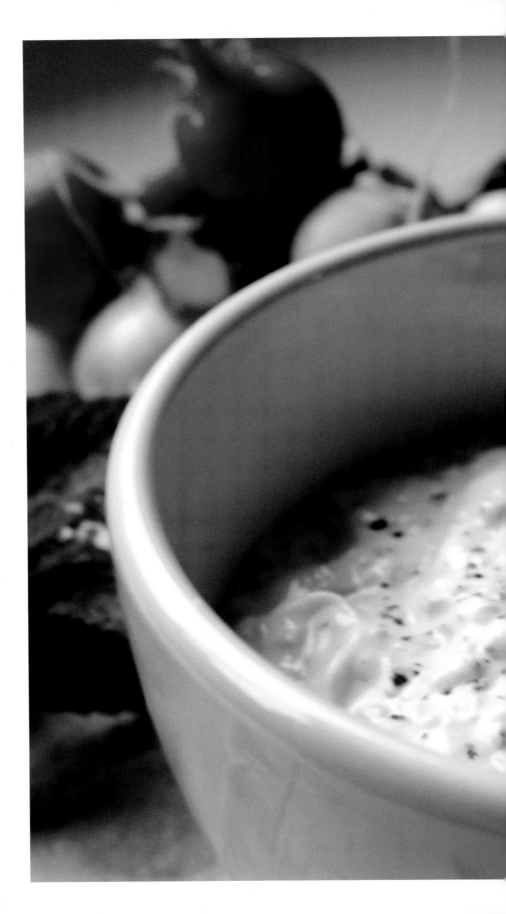

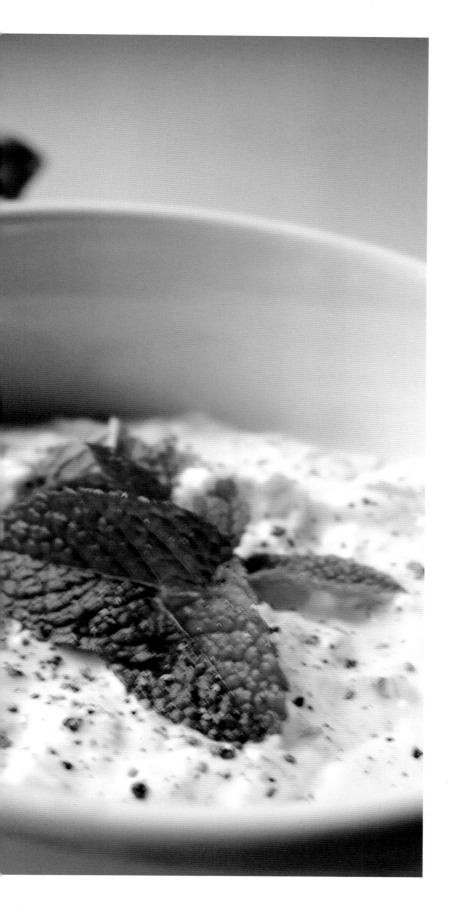

Radish Tzatziki with Veggie Sticks

MAKES ABOUT 3 CUPS

Keeps up to 3 days in the fridge.

You will need a grater or a food processor.

5 radishes, quartered
1 Lebanese cucumber, chopped
200–300ml natural Greek yoghurt
juice of ½ a lemon
rind of ½ a lemon
3 tbsp extra virgin olive oil
generous pinch of salt
mint to garnish
cracked pepper to garnish

❶ Grate the radish and cucumber, or you can use a food processor to roughly chop them. Strain away any excess liquid. Place in a bowl, add yoghurt and combine.

❷ Add lemon juice, rind, olive oil and salt and mix well. If the dip is too runny—add a touch more yoghurt.

❸ Garnish with mint and cracked pepper to serve.

LUNCH

Just like breakfast, your lunch should contain good-quality proteins and fats. Breakfast and lunch should be the larger meals of the day, to take the pressure off dinner. You will sleep better at night after a light meal.

Spiced and Roasted Pumpkin Soup

SERVES 4

You will need a medium baking dish and a handheld or bench-top blender.

½ medium pumpkin (whichever variety you prefer)

olive oil

salt and pepper to taste

1 onion, chopped

3 parsnips, peeled and chopped

2 carrots, peeled and chopped

6 cups vegetable stock

1 tsp dried chilli

½ cup your preferred milk (or cream)

1 tsp cinnamon

❶ Preheat oven to 200°C. Peel, de-seed and chop the pumpkin into chunks. Place in a bowl, drizzle with olive oil, season with salt and pepper and toss for an even coverage. Add to a baking dish and bake in the oven for 30 minutes or until well roasted— it can be slightly brown at the edges.

❷ Meanwhile, heat a little olive oil in a large pot. Add onion, parsnip and carrot, and fry over a medium heat until cooked.

❸ Add pumpkin, stock and chilli and allow to simmer for at least 30 minutes. In the final stages, add milk. Blend well and season to taste. Serve with a sprinkling of cinnamon.

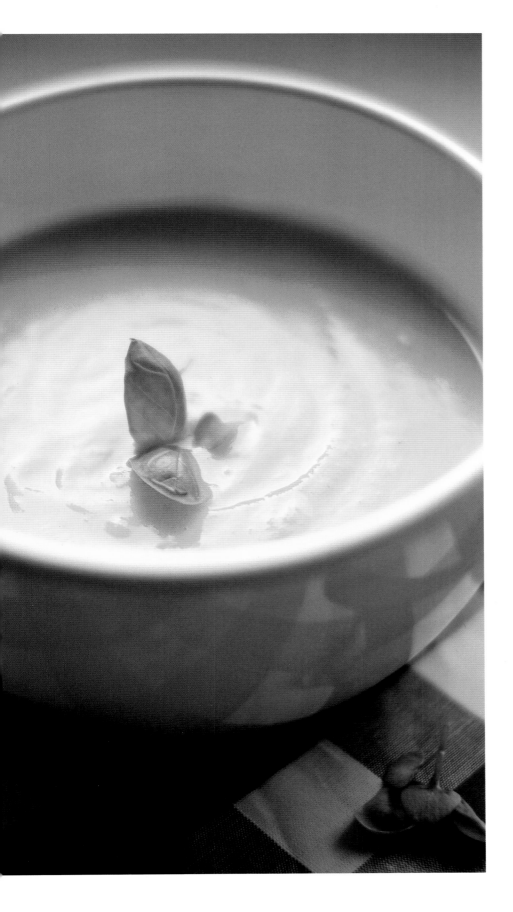

Mango Salsa Cups

SERVES 2

You will just need a salad bowl.

1 mango, finely chopped
½ red onion, diced
1 small bunch of coriander
   (or parsley), chopped
½ avocado, diced
2 celery sticks, finely diced
juice of ½ a lemon
dash of olive oil
salt and pepper
1 endive, pulled apart

❶ Combine mango, onion,
   coriander, avocado, celery,
   lemon juice and olive oil.

❷ Season with salt and pepper
   to taste and mix well.

❸ Spoon mixture into the
   separated leaves of the
   endive and serve.

Bean Salad

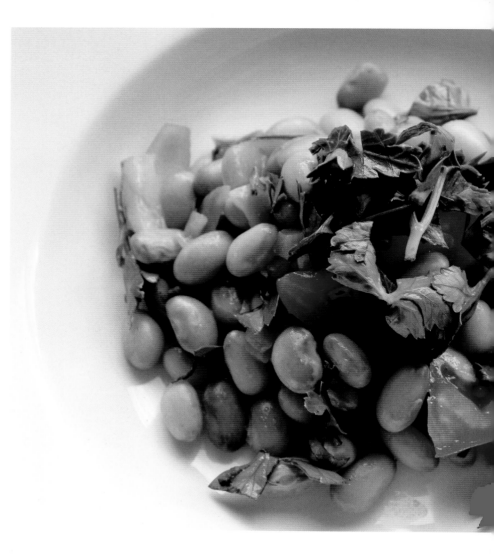

SERVES 2

You will need a medium saucepan.

2 tbsp coconut oil

2 bay leaves

1 red onion, finely sliced

1½ cups dried borlotti beans,
   soaked

2–3 tomatoes

½ bunch parsley,
   roughly chopped

2 tbsp apple cider vinegar

2 tbsp olive oil

salt and pepper

❶ Heat coconut oil in your saucepan over a medium heat, add the bay
leaves and half the red onion and allow to soften. Add the beans and
just enough water to cover them. Simmer for at least twenty minutes,
until the beans are cooked.

❷ Meanwhile, dice the tomatoes and place in a salad bowl with parsley,
remaining red onion, vinegar, olive oil and salt and pepper. Mix well
to allow juices to combine.

❸ When the beans are done, drain and allow to cool. Combine with
tomatoes, mix well and serve.

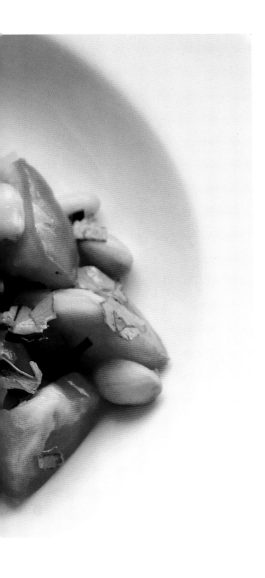

Baked Potatoes with Coleslaw

Using organic carrots and apples means you can eat the skin, a good source of nutrients.

SERVES 2

4 small baking potatoes

½ white cabbage

1 organic carrot

1 organic apple

3 tbsp olive oil

2 tbsp apple cider vinegar

salt and pepper

❶ Preheat oven to 220°C. Bake potatoes for 40 minutes, or until cooked through.

❷ Meanwhile, shred cabbage by slicing very finely. Grate carrot and apple with the skin on and add to the cabbage, tossing to combine. Combine 2 tbsp olive oil with apple cider and salt and pepper and pour over coleslaw.

❸ When cooked, break the skin of the potatoes, drizzle with remaining olive oil and season with salt and pepper. Serve together with coleslaw.

Rocket, Pea and Currant Salad

SERVES 4

1 bag of rocket, washed
1 bunch of parsley, chopped
1 cup of cooked peas
⅓ cup of currants
3 spring onions, chopped
olive oil
fresh lemon juice
salt and pepper to season
raspberries to garnish

❶ Combine rocket, parsley, peas and currants in a large salad bowl.

❷ Drizzle with oil, lemon juice, salt and pepper to taste, before tossing salad.

❸ Garnish with raspberries and serve.

Avocado, Walnut and Pear Salad

SERVES 1

You will need a salad spinner and a clean jam jar with a fitted lid.

Use activated nuts if possible (see Snacks).

1 large handful salad mix, washed and spun
½ avocado, sliced
10–12 walnuts, crumbled
½ pear thinly sliced
¼ red onion, thinly sliced
5–6 leaves basil or mint, chopped

DRESSING
2 tbsp olive oil
2 tbsp apple cider vinegar
½ clove of garlic, crushed

❶ Combine salad ingredients in a serving bowl.

❷ For the dressing, combine ingredients in a jar. Screw on the lid nice and tight, and shake vigorously until creamy. Pour over salad and serve immediately.

Broad Bean and Pomegranate Salad

If broad beans are in season, I like to use the fresh variety. Otherwise, you'll find them near the peas in the freezer section of your supermarket.

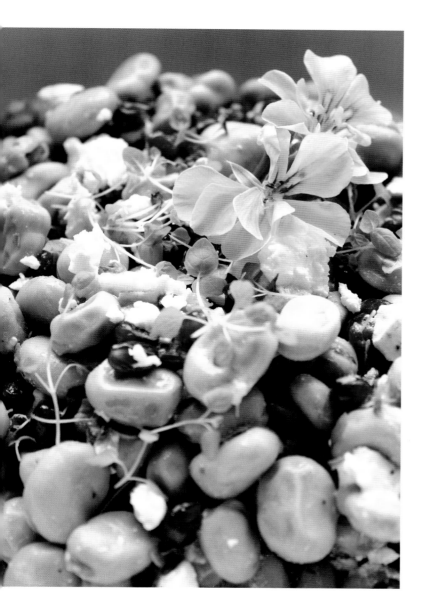

SERVES 4

You will need a clean jam jar with a fitted lid.

200g broad beans, cooked

seeds of 1 pomegranate

1 jar Persian feta

½ bunch mint, finely chopped

juice of 1 lemon

1 clove garlic, crushed

3 tbsp olive oil

salt and pepper

❶ In a salad bowl, place broad beans, pomegranate, feta (reserving a little to serve) and half the mint.

❷ In your jar, combine lemon, crushed garlic, oil, salt and pepper—screw on the lid nice and tight, and shake vigorously until creamy. Pour dressing over the salad and toss to coat.

❸ Garnish with remaining feta and mint and serve.

Cauliflower Soup

SERVES 4

You will need a large stock pot or saucepan and a handheld or bench-top blender.

⅓ **cup olive oil or coconut oil**

2 onions, roughly chopped

3 garlic cloves, roughly chopped

1 medium-sized cauliflower, in florets

5 cups stock (I use vegetable, mum uses chicken)

1 cup your preferred milk (or cream)

crusty bread to serve

1 Heat oil in your pot, add onion and garlic and cook for 3–4 minutes until glossy.

2 Add cauliflower and cook until it begins to brown. Cover with stock and bring it to the boil. Reduce heat and cook for at least 30 minutes (the longer the better).

3 Blend until you reach a very smooth consistency. Add the milk and combine well.

4 Serve with crusty bread.

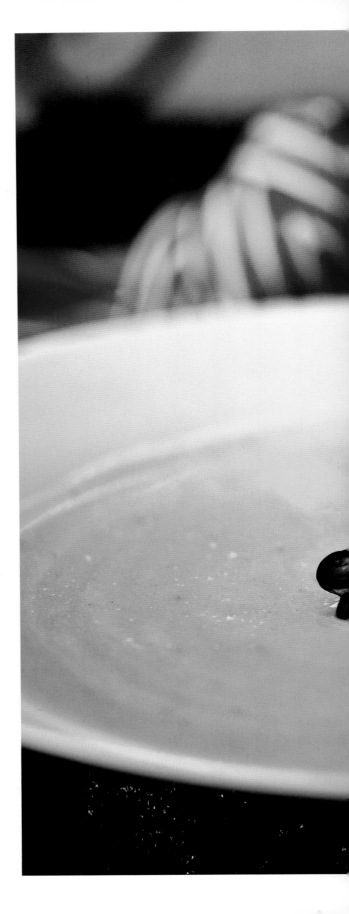

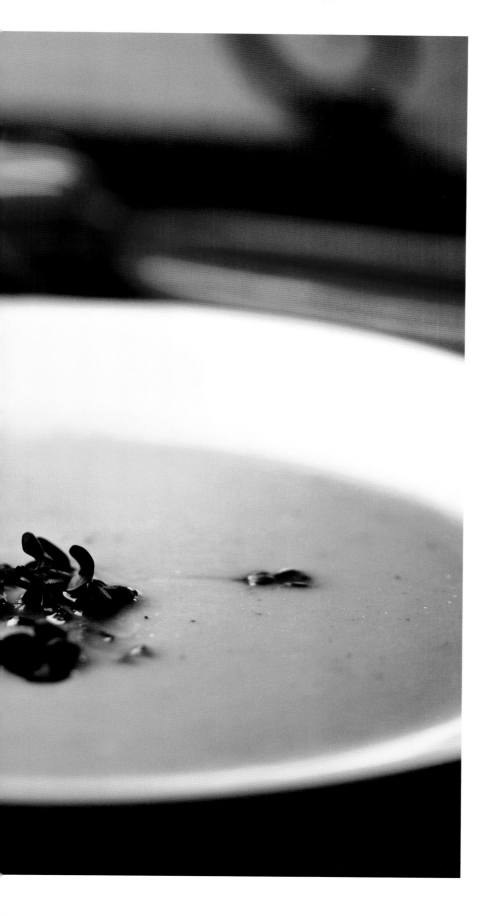

Lentil and Haloumi Salad

SERVES 2

You will need a fry pan.

3 tomatoes, diced
1 red onion, thinly sliced
handful mint, chopped (reserve
    two sprigs to garnish)
salt and pepper
1 tbsp olive oil, plus extra to drizzle
250g haloumi
1½ cups cooked lentils
    (or one can)

❶ Mix the tomatoes with the red
   onion, mint and salt and pepper
   and then set aside.

❷ Heat olive oil in your fry pan over
   a medium heat. Slice haloumi
   into 1cm slices and fry until
   golden on each side.

❸ Combine lentils and tomato
   mixture, drizzle with olive oil and
   top with haloumi and mint sprigs
   to serve.

DINNER

Dinner will ideally be the smallest meal of the day to allow your body to rest and rejuvenate overnight. As we know, sleep is important for healthy hormones—allow the gut to repair during the night rather than digest.

Grilled Veggie Stacks

SERVES 2

You will need a pastry brush.

Add your favourite vegetables to the stack.

You can also serve with Homemade Pesto (see Snacks).

1 medium sweet potato
1 eggplant
2 Roma tomatoes
2 tbsp olive oil
salt and pepper
handful basil leaves

❶ Preheat oven to 200°C. Peel sweet potato and cut into ½cm slices, discarding the narrow ends. Brush with oil and arrange on a baking tray. Cut eggplant into 1cm slices, brush with oil and arrange on a separate tray. Cut tomatoes lengthwise and add to one of the trays. Bake veggies for at least 30 minutes, or until beginning to brown.

❷ Season with salt and pepper and layer veggies onto two dinner plates. Drizzle with olive oil, garnish with basil leaves and serve.

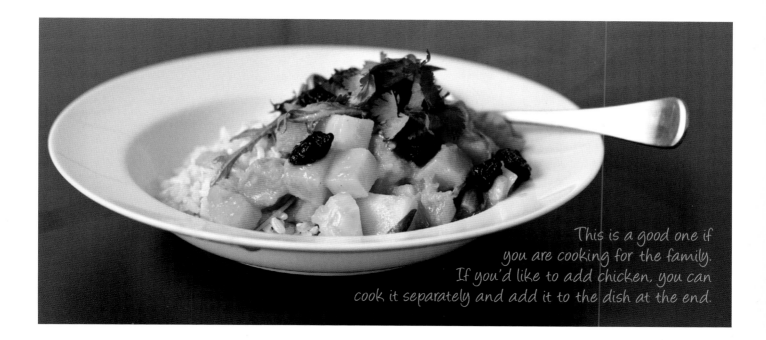

This is a good one if
you are cooking for the family.
If you'd like to add chicken, you can
cook it separately and add it to the dish at the end.

Pumpkin Curry

SERVES 4

You will need a large, deep fry pan or a medium saucepan.

1 tbsp coconut oil for frying

2 tbsp red curry paste (try to
   avoid versions with added
   sugar and preservatives)

1 clove garlic, crushed

1 onion, chopped

½ butternut pumpkin,
   in 2cm cubes

2 potatoes, in 2cm cubes

4 dates, roughly chopped

1 can coconut milk (full cream)

1 red capsicum, deseeded

1 bunch spinach or similar greens

salt and pepper

2 cups brown rice, cooked, to serve

❶ Heat coconut oil in your fry pan or saucepan over a medium heat. Add curry paste and heat for 2 minutes until fragrant. Add garlic and onion and stir. Add pumpkin, potato, dates, coconut milk and a small amount of water (about ¼ cup).

❷ Cover and allow to cook until pumpkin becomes soft.

❸ Cut capsicum into strips and add to mixture. Cook for a further 3–4 minutes before adding spinach.

❹ Season with salt and pepper and serve with brown rice.

Stuffed Capsicums

SERVES 2

You will need a medium fry pan.

2 tbsp coconut oil or olive oil

1 onion, finely chopped

5–6 mushrooms, finely sliced

½ cup peas, fresh or frozen

1 cup cooked white or brown rice

few sprigs thyme

salt and pepper

2 medium capsicums

❶ Preheat oven to 200°C. Heat 1 tablespoon of oil in fry pan over a medium heat. Fry onion until clear. Add mushrooms and peas and sauté until peas are tender and mushrooms are lightly browned. Add rice and thyme and season with salt and pepper. Stir until hot and well combined. Set aside.

❷ Slice the stalk top off each capsicum and discard. Remove the seeds and pith from the capsicum. Fill each empty shell with rice mixture and drizzle with remaining oil.

❸ Bake for 20 minutes or until the capsicum no longer resists a knife or skewer. Serve with a green salad.

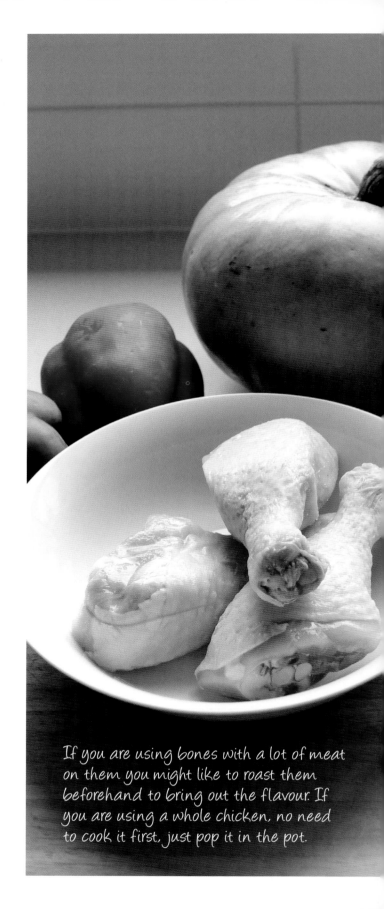

If you are using bones with a lot of meat on them you might like to roast them beforehand to bring out the flavour. If you are using a whole chicken, no need to cook it first, just pop it in the pot.

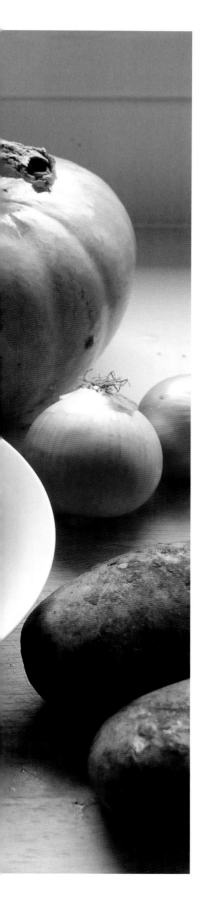

Beautiful Bone Broth

Bone broth is one of the most healing recipes on the planet! It goes to work on your digestive system, pumps up your vitamin and mineral tanks and can be consumed as is or used as stock for other soups and stews. I suggest making up a big batch (this recipe makes 3 litres) and freezing into ice-cube trays to have on hand at any time. I've been known to ask patients to switch their arvo cuppa for a cup of bone broth. It can also be a gentle transition food for vegetarians who have decided to reincorporate meat protein into their diet. The amino acids found in meat are a great way to balance out hormones.

MAKES 3 LITRES

You will need a large stock pot.

1 large chicken or 2kg of bones (beef ribs, neck or shoulder bones—ask your butcher for soup bones)

1 cup apple cider vinegar

3 carrots, finely chopped

3 celery sticks, finely chopped

a few sprigs thyme and parsley, tied together

salt and pepper

❶ Place bones and vinegar in a large pot, add enough water to cover and allow it to sit for an hour or so.

❷ Drain the bones, then add them with the carrot, celery, herbs and seasoning to the pot with 3 litres of water. Bring to the boil, and then reduce to a simmer for at least 2 hours. The longer this cooks, the better.

❸ Remove the herb bundle before serving or storing.

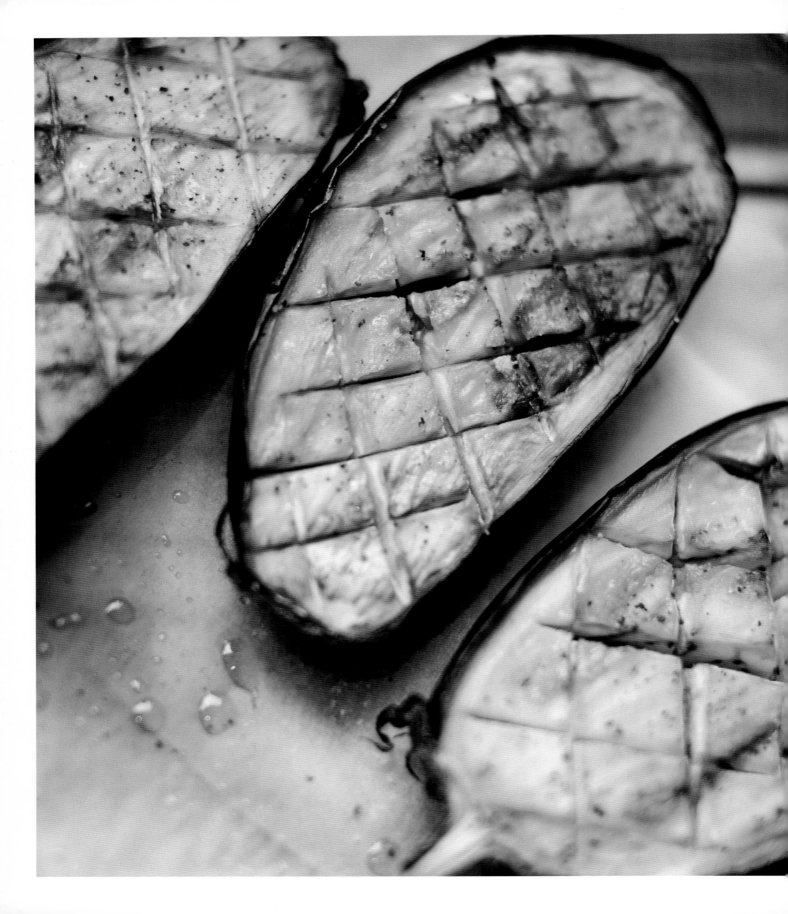

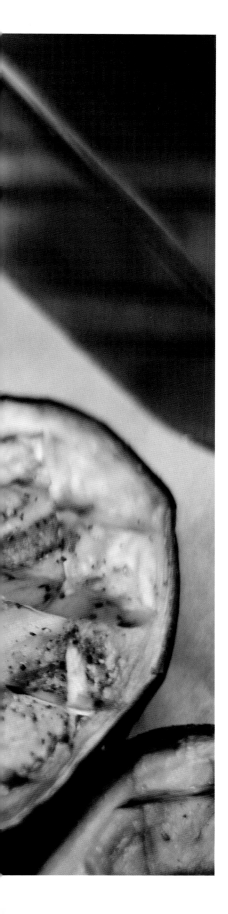

Stuffed Eggplant

You could top this with feta or goat's cheese before putting into the oven for extra flavour. Or, for a meat variety, add chicken mince to the onions, cook through before adding tomatoes.

SERVES 2

You will need a baking tray.

2 larger eggplants

1 tbsp your preferred oil for frying, plus extra for eggplant

2 onions, chopped

1 can organic, crushed tomatoes

salt and pepper

1 bunch parsley

1. Preheat oven to 180°C. Cut the eggplant in half, score and brush with oil. Bake until flesh is soft, approximately 30 minutes. Remove from oven and allow to cool enough for easy handling.

2. Meanwhile, heat oil in a pan and fry onion until soft. Add tomato and salt and pepper and stir.

3. Remove the flesh from the eggplant halves by scoring around the edge, leaving a 0.5cm border, and then spooning it out carefully, trying to keep the shape of the skins intact, as they are to be stuffed. Add the eggplant flesh and parsley to the tomatoes and stir to combine.

4. Place mixture back into eggplant skins and pop back into the oven for approximately 10 minutes.

Mexican Feast

SERVES 4

You will need a food processor, a large saucepan, a large baking tray and a medium-sized fry pan.

CORN CHOWDER

cooked kernels of 5 corn cobs

3 spring onions

35g semolina

1L hot vegetable stock

150g plain tortilla chips

75g grated cheese

½ bunch coriander, picked

❶ Preheat oven to 200°C. Place corn kernels into a food processor with spring onions and semolina. Blitz until mushy.

❷ Transfer the mixture into your saucepan, add the hot stock and bring to the boil, then turn it down and let it simmer for 10 minutes.

❸ Meanwhile, spread out the tortilla chips on your foil-lined baking tray and sprinkle with cheese. Warm for 5–10 minutes until the cheese melts.

❹ Serve soup into bowls and decorate with a few cheese chips on each. Reserve the remaining chips. Sprinkle soup with coriander and serve immediately.

AVOCADO GUACAMOLE

2 ripe avocados

1 cup sour cream

2 spring onions

salt and pepper

❶ Combine all ingredients in a food processor until smooth. Serve with cheese chips (see Corn Chowder above).

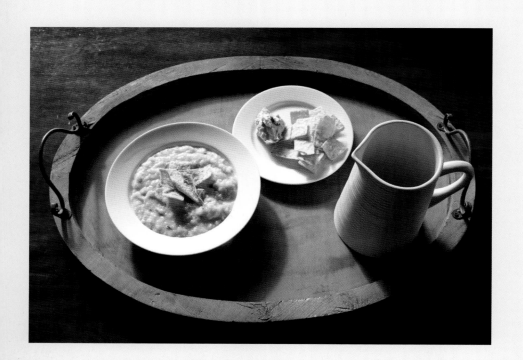

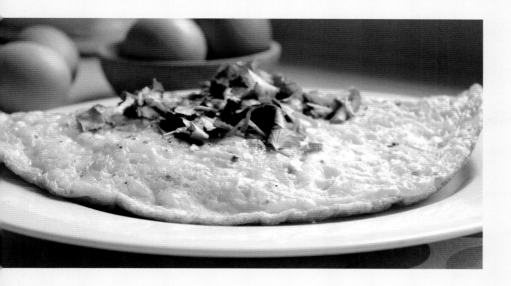

MEXICAN OMELETTE

4 eggs
⅓ cup your preferred milk
¾ cup of grated cheese
salt and pepper
1 tbsp coconut oil
½ red capsicum, chopped
2 spring onions, chopped
¼ cup parsley, chopped

❶ Whisk eggs together. Add milk, cheese, salt and pepper and combine well.

❷ Heat coconut oil in your fry pan. Pour in egg mixture and allow to cook for 2 minutes on a medium heat.

❸ Sprinkle over capsicum, onion and parsley and cook for a further minute.

❹ Turn out and cut into strips or quarters to serve. Garnish with parsley.

BEAN AND TUNA FRITTERS

1 cup cooked or canned beans
1 can quality tuna or similar
**   quantity fresh fish, cooked**
4 large potatoes, peeled,
**   steamed and mashed**
30g rice flour
1 egg
½ bunch parsley
2 spring onions, chopped
salt and pepper
approx. ⅔ cup oil for frying
lemon to serve

❶ Add all ingredients except oil and lemon into a bowl and combine.

❷ Pour enough oil to reach about 1cm in a fry pan and get it hot enough that a drop of water sizzles on contact. Maintaining a medium heat, with two tablespoons, scoop out batter to fill one spoon and use the other to gently drop the mixture into the oil. Flatten the fritters gently with a fork, leaving at least 1cm space between each one. Fry for 2–3 minutes on each side or until light brown.

❸ Place fritters on paper towel to absorb excess oil. Serve with lemon wedges and a big green salad.

SERIOUSLY AWESOME SALSA

3 tomatoes, diced
½ bunch spring onions, chopped
2 avocados, chopped
**   (reserve pits)**
1 bunch coriander
juice of 1 lemon
salt, pepper and oil to season

❶ Combine ingredients and seasoning in a bowl. Place the avocado seeds in the mixture to prevent the avocado from going brown. Cover and let sit for 30 minutes to allow juices to combine. Remove the avocado seeds before serving.

Spinach and Ricotta Pie

So simple. If you're adventurous you can experiment by adding mushrooms to the filling, or pine nuts to the top of the pie.

SERVES 6

You will need a deep-sided, ovenproof dish, such as a flan or pie dish.

BASE

2 cups cooked brown rice

40g butter, melted

2 egg yolks (reserve whites for pie filling)

FILLING

500ml ricotta

2 eggs

½ tsp nutmeg

salt and pepper

2 bunches spinach or 1 bunch silverbeet, washed

❶ Preheat oven to 200°C.

❷ To make the base, mix together rice, butter and egg yolks.

❸ Grease your pie dish and press the base mixture firmly down into the bottom of the dish. Bake in the oven for approximately 15 minutes or until it begins to brown.

❹ Meanwhile, make the filling. Place ricotta into a bowl and soften it using a potato masher. Add eggs, reserved egg whites, nutmeg and salt and pepper and combine well. Chop spinach or silverbeet into 1cm strips and combine with the ricotta mixture. Scoop onto rice base and bake for 20 minutes or until top begins to brown.

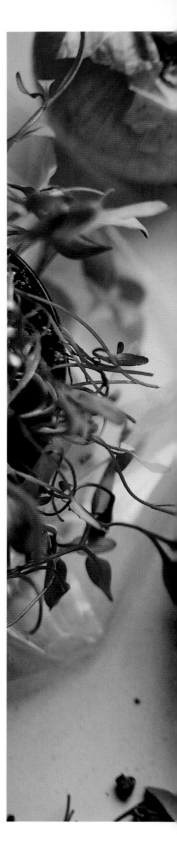

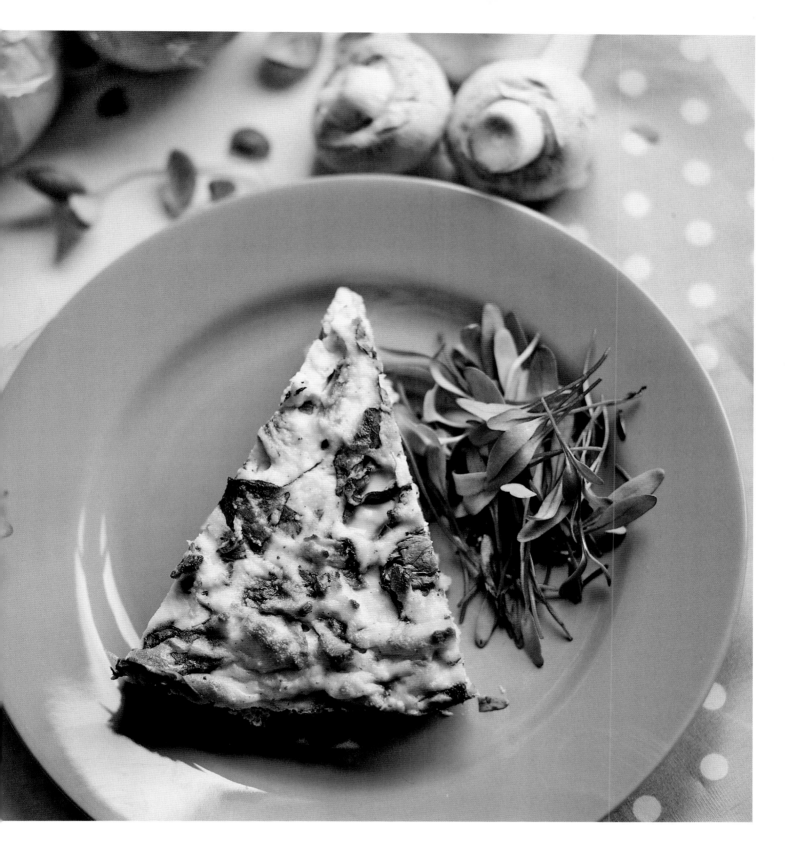

DESSERTS

You can have your cake and eat it too! It's all about using whole foods to maximise digestion.

Moist Cocoa Cake

MAKES 1 CAKE

You will need a springform cake tin and an electric mixer.

1½ cups rice flour

1½ tbsp baking powder

1½ tsp bicarb soda

½ teaspoon salt

3 eggs

½ cup coconut butter, melted

1 cup xylitol (dextrose)

½ cup cold, organic decaffeinated
   coffee

¾ cup yoghurt

½ cup cocoa

seeds of 1 vanilla bean

ICING

1 tsp cocoa

2 tbsp xylitol

1–2 tbsp coconut oil, melted

❶ Preheat oven to 180°C. Grease and line your cake tin. Sift dry ingredients together. Mix wet ingredients together and add to dries, beating with an electric mixer until thoroughly combined.

❷ Pour mix into prepared tin and bake for about 30 minutes or until a skewer inserted in the middle comes out clean. Cool on a wire rack.

❸ To ice, place the cake back into the tin to avoid drips. Combine the cocoa and xylitol well. Brush top of cake generously with coconut oil and use a sifter to cover with cocoa mixture. Allow to set.

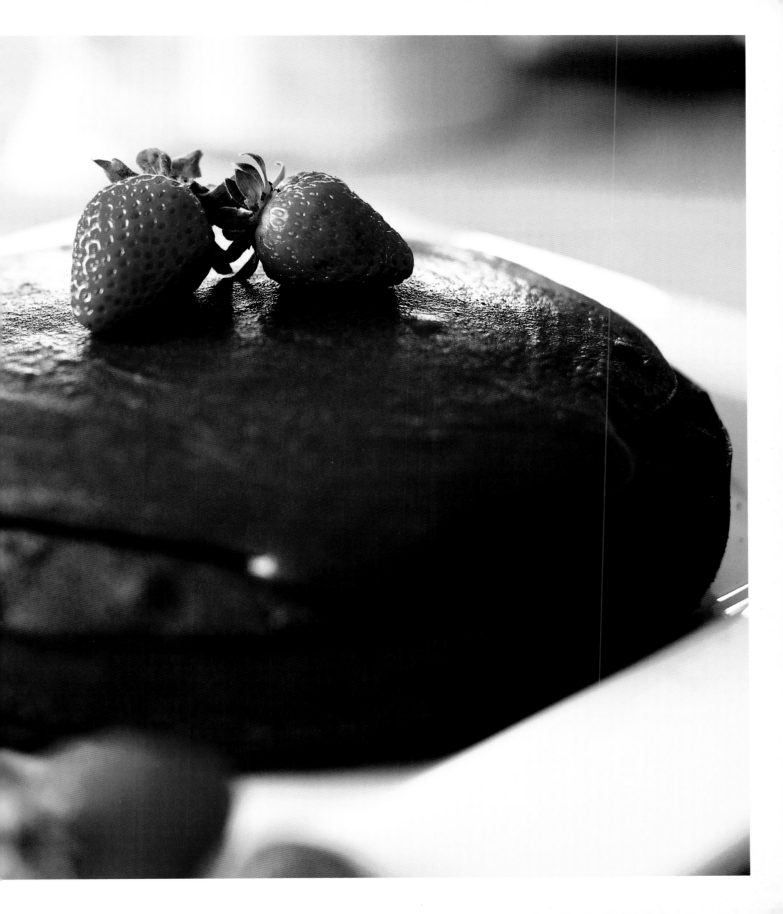

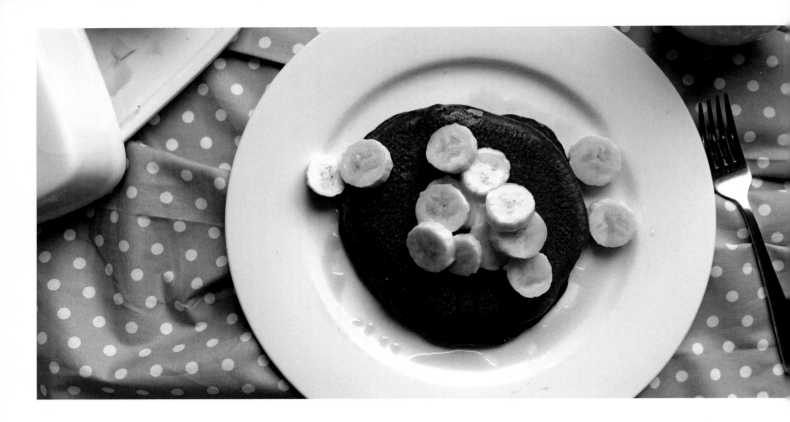

Buckwheat Pancakes

SERVES 4

You will need a handheld or electric egg beater and a fry pan.

3 eggs
180g buckwheat flour
170ml your preferred milk
1 heaped tsp baking soda
pinch of salt
knob of butter for frying

1 Separate eggs, placing yolks into a larger bowl. Add flour, milk and baking soda to the yolks and combined well, until a smooth batter forms.

2 Add a pinch of salt to the egg whites and beat until they form stiff peaks. Using a wooden spoon, fold egg whites into the batter to combine.

3 Heat butter in a fry pan. Add a quarter of the batter and cook pancake, turning when bubbles rise to the surface. Repeat until all four pancakes are cooked.

4 Enjoy with fruit and yoghurt or, for a savoury pancake, add corn kernels to the batter just before flipping.

Beanielicious Brownies

MAKES 1 TRAY

You will need a good brownie tray.

½ cup cooked or canned
    white beans
250g dark chocolate
125g organic, unsalted butter
1 cup walnuts, chopped
½ cup coconut flour
pinch of salt
4 eggs

❶ Preheat oven to 180°C. Grease and line your brownie tray.

❷ Puree beans using a blender or food processor until a smooth paste forms. Set aside.

❸ Melt chocolate and butter and combine. (Alternatively, reserve half the chocolate and chop it into chunks to add to the batter, for a chocolate-chip effect.)

❹ To the bean puree add walnuts, coconut flour, salt and chocolate mixture and stir until roughly combined. In a separate bowl, beat eggs for about a minute—until light and fluffy. Fold through bean batter (you would add chocolate chunks here).

❺ Pour into prepared tray and spread evenly and bake for 30 minutes or until just cooked through. Remove from oven and allow to cool.

❻ Cut into slices and dust with cocoa to serve.

Tropical Tapioca Pudding with Mango Coulis

SERVES 6

You will need a small saucepan, a silicone muffin tray or 6 small jelly moulds and 6 parfait glasses, martini glasses or other attractive serving glasses.

PUDDING

1 cup tapioca

6 cups water

seeds of 1 vanilla bean

1 can organic coconut cream

coconut oil to grease moulds

mint to garnish

COULIS AND GARNISH

2 mangoes, sliced

¼ cup water

1. Combine tapioca, water and vanilla in saucepan and bring to the boil. Simmer for 10–15 minutes (no longer) until the tapioca is almost clear. Allow it to set overnight.

2. The next day, rinse the cooked tapioca under cold water and place it in a bowl, combining with 1 cup of the coconut cream.

3. Prepare moulds by greasing with coconut oil. Spoon in tapioca mixture and pop into fridge to set.

4. For the coulis, add one half of the sliced mango to your saucepan with water. Stir over a low to medium heat until it reaches the consistency of jam—approximately 10 minutes. Allow to cool.

5. Spoon mango coulis evenly into serving glasses. Turn out individual tapioca puddings over the top and set aside, allowing them to come back to room temperature.

6. Warm the remaining coconut cream. Pour around the pudding, sharing evenly between glasses.

7. Garnish with remaining mango slices and mint.

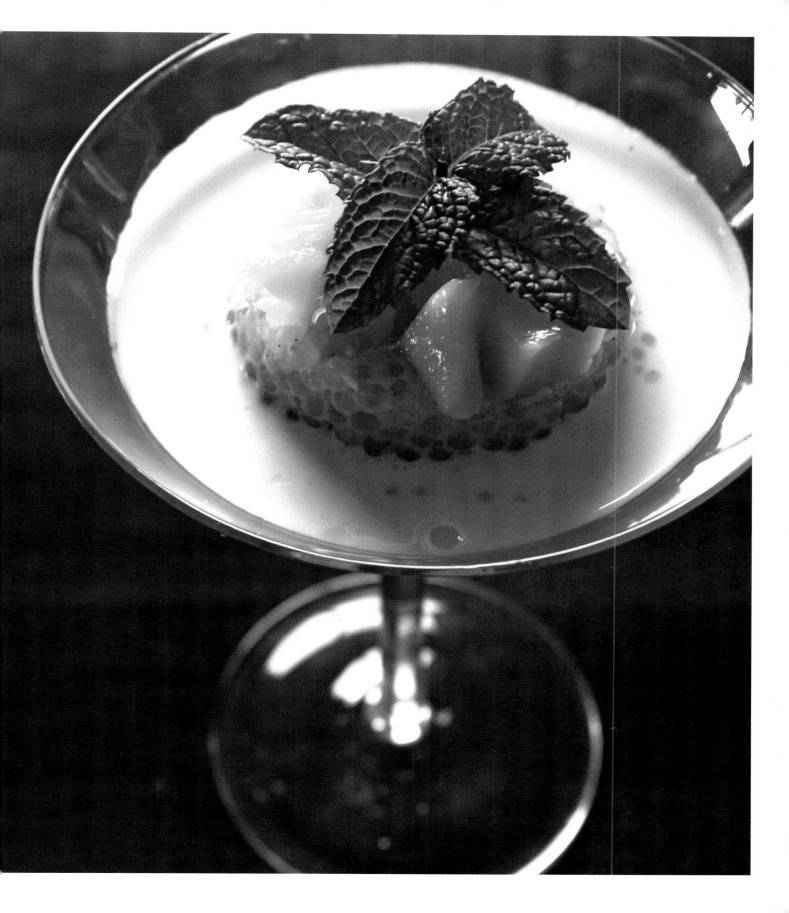

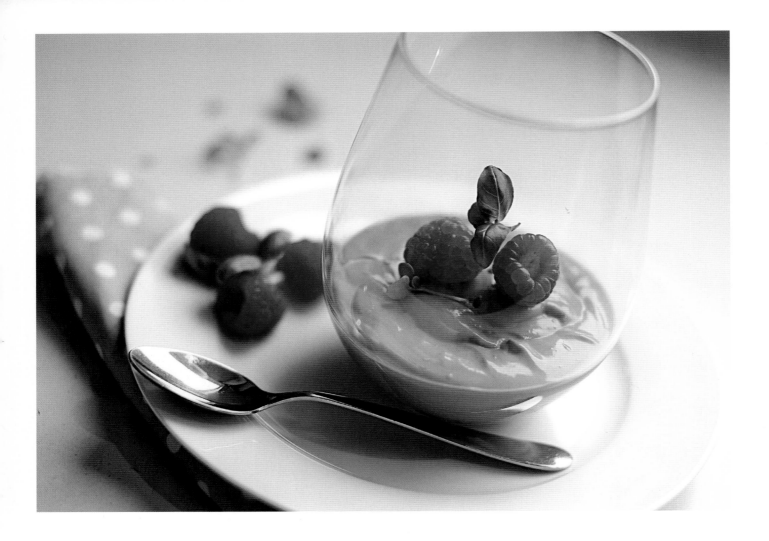

Chocolate Mousse

If you search for dark chocolate without any milk solids, this mousse can be entirely vegan.

SERVES 4

You will need a handheld blender or electric mixer.

200ml coconut cream

250g dark chocolate, melted,
   plus extra 40g to serve

2 tsp pure maple syrup

2 tsp peanut butter

❶ Blend all ingredients, except extra chocolate, until just smooth, without over mixing. Pour into small dishes or glasses. Refrigerate for at least 2 hours until set.

❷ Grate extra chocolate and sprinkle over to serve.

Raspberry Moulds
with Lemon Balm and Double Cream

SERVES 2

You will need a small saucepan and two small jelly moulds.
Lemon balm can be substituted with mint if unavailable.

4 punnets fresh raspberries or two cups frozen
1 bunch lemon balm, finely chopped
½ cup honey
1 sachet gelatin
double cream to serve

❶ In a saucepan, combine raspberries, ¾ of the
lemon balm and honey over a very low heat
for roughly 10 minutes. Once the berries have
broken down, push mixture through a sieve
to remove raspberry seeds.

❷ In a clean saucepan, stir mixture continuously
over a medium heat—never quite allowing it
to boil. When near boiling, sprinkle gelatin
over the top and stir well until dissolved. Pour
into your moulds and refrigerate for 2 hours
or until set.

❸ Turn out and garnish with cream and remaining
lemon balm.

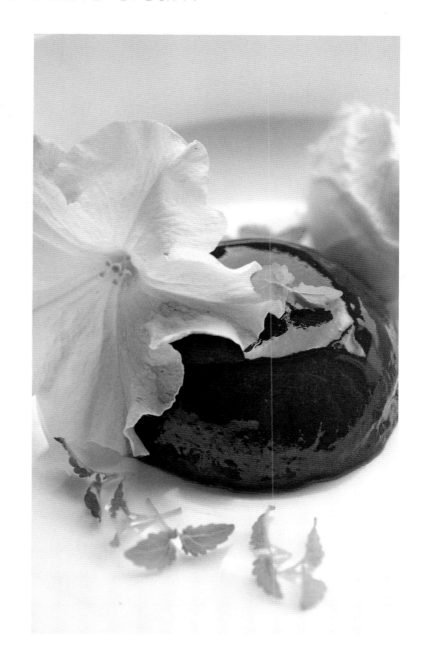

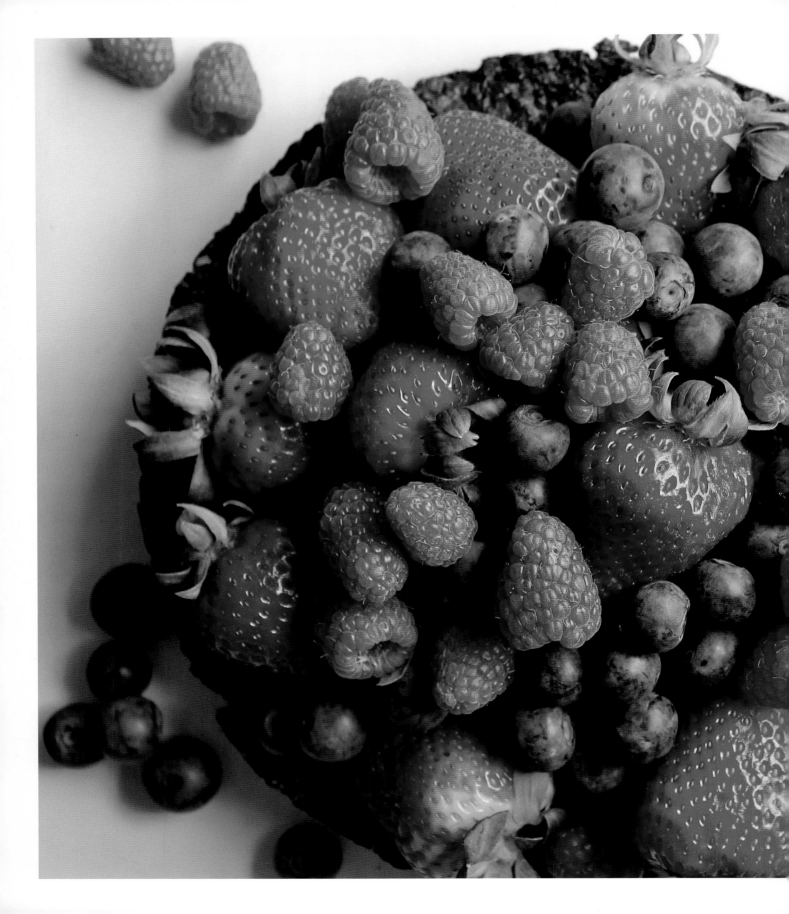

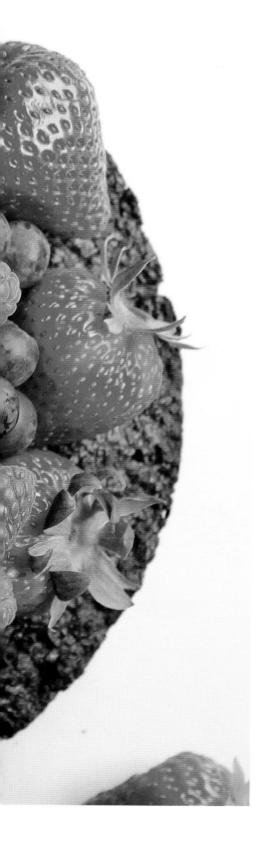

Chocolate Torte with Berries

MAKES 1 TORTE

You will need a spring-form cake tin, a food processor and a handheld or electric egg beater. You can serve once cool but it is best if refrigerated overnight.

250g roasted almonds

250g quality dark chocolate (the more cocoa content, the better)

125g dates

125g dried figs

6 egg whites

1 cup berries and whipped cream to serve

1 Preheat oven to 180°C. Grease and line your cake tin.

2 In a food processor, chop almonds and chocolate roughly.

3 Chop dates and figs by hand.

4 Beat egg whites until stiff. Fold almonds, chocolate and fruit into the egg whites and transfer the mixture into your cake tin. Bake for 45 minutes. Then, turn the heat off, open the oven door slightly and allow the torte to cool in the tin.

5 Turn out onto a platter and refrigerate overnight.

6 Decorate with berries and serve with a dollop of cream!

DRINKS

Your body will love you for warm drinks. Cool drinks are not bad for you, but just make sure they aren't taken on an empty stomach, and try to avoid ice-cold drinks.

My clients enjoy green tea, ground-bean coffee—one per day is enough and not too much—herbal tisanes, black leaf teas and nut milk. Kombucha (fermented tea), homemade or from your health-food shop, can also be heated up.

First thing in the morning, a cold drink on an empty stomach delivers a shock to the digestive system. Grab a glass of warm water instead.

Nut Milk

Nut milk is super easy to make and equally easy for your gut to digest.

MAKES ABOUT ½ LITRE
You will need a handheld or bench-top blender and a piece of cheesecloth or muslin.
It will last for 2 days in the fridge.

1 cup organic nuts of your choice
2 cups water
your preferred sweetener (optional)

❶ Soak nuts in water overnight or up to 2 days.

❷ Strain off liquid (it will look milky) and set aside. Rinse off the nuts (they will feel squishy). Combine nuts and liquid and blend for 2 minutes. Pour the milk through a strainer—you'll be left with what resembles almond meal. Strain the meal through a piece of cheesecloth or muslin, adding the liquid to the milk and discarding the meal (unless you want to use it).

❸ Sweeten if desired. Serve!

Cocao Cocoa

Do you own a coffee machine? If you do, simply heat up a cup of milk using the milk nozzle and add 2 teaspoons of cocao. If not, heat the milk gently in a saucepan on the stove instead, and whisk in the cocao at the end. I realise unsweetened cocao isn't everybody's cup of tea, so you can of course sweeten it to your liking. If you are cutting out sugar, try xylitol or stevia.

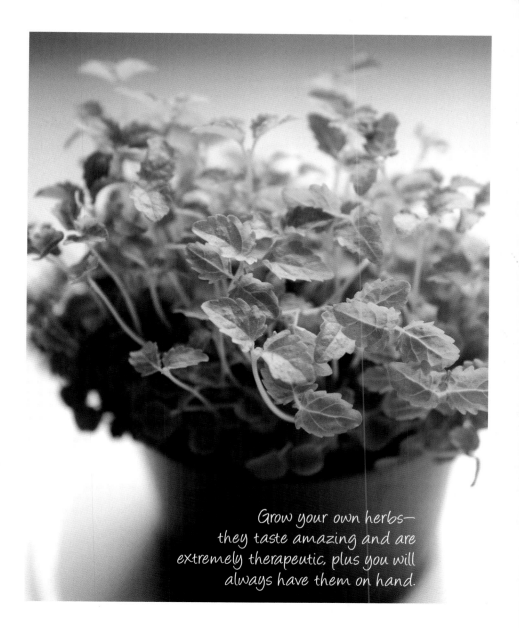

Grow your own herbs—
they taste amazing and are
extremely therapeutic, plus you will
always have them on hand.

Out and About?

No problem—you can always find a healthy, fertile option. When all else fails, make eggs your go-to meal—readily available at any time of the day.

At sandwich bars ask for a plate of salad and cold meats. Be mindful that sauces and dressings can be high in sugar. A better option is to dress your salads with some oil and lemon juice or vinegar.

In winter, soups and stews are perfect, just as a salad with some protein is in summer.

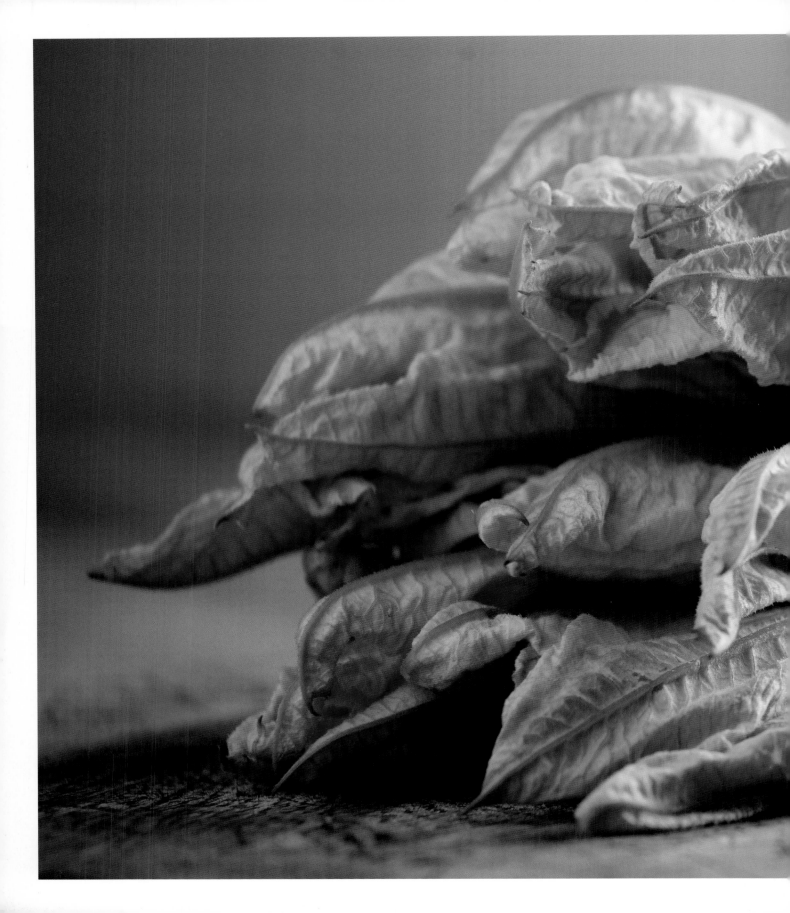

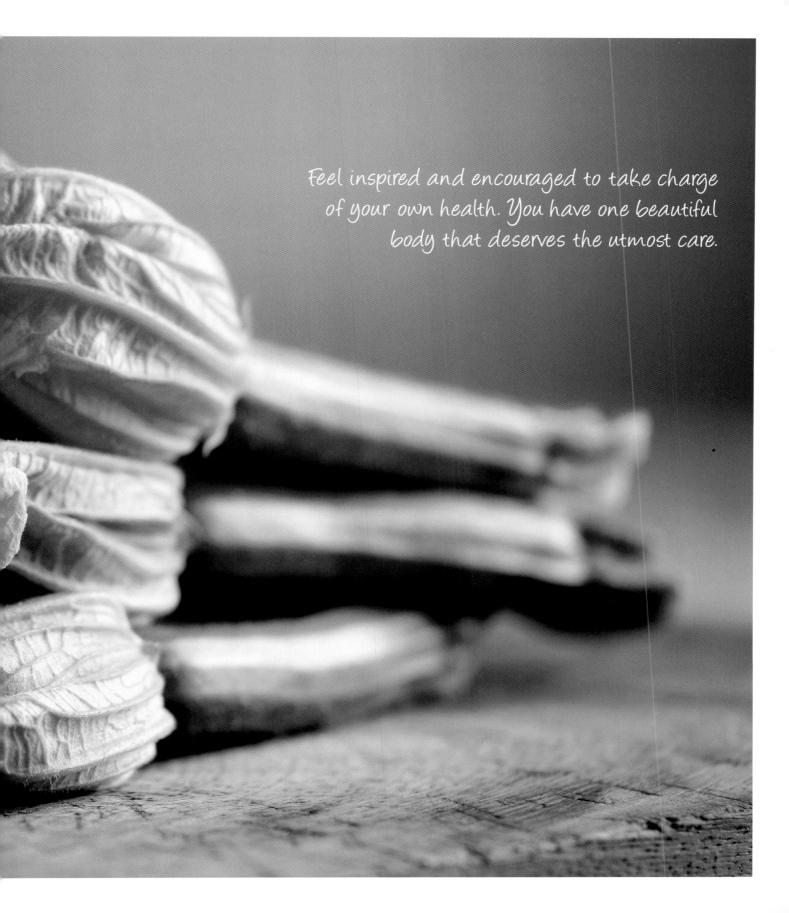

Feel inspired and encouraged to take charge of your own health. You have one beautiful body that deserves the utmost care.

CONCLUSION

*Y*ou now have all you need to get your health and hormones firing! Remember, while fertility will give you the potential to conceive, it's not just about babies, it's a way to live.

All of us, whether couples or singles, benefit from eating toward fertility and happy hormones. Sometimes fertility is complicated, and due to the stresses of our environment and a myriad of other influences, we can get the sense that it's out of our hands. Taking control of the things that we can influence is therefore paramount.

Perhaps you're still young and babies are not on your to-do list. Either way, I encourage you to be inspired, maintaining fertility for when the time is right for you. The consolation prize is your maximum health and vitality, a healthier menstrual cycle, and a very happy digestive system.

Maybe you've been trying for a baby for a very long time. Eating for fertility and improving your body's overall wellness, not least your emotional health, can increase the chance of successful conception by up to 50%. Consuming the right kind of food is a no brainer, and something you can start to implement today.

If you were to fall pregnant tomorrow, I know you would want the best possible start for your baby's life. With this book I hope to enable in you the gift of wellness and a heightened awareness of your body and how it communicates with you. Use it to live a fertile life.

Fertility remains relevant through the post-reproductive life phases, as it extends through to healthy loving relationships and emotional wellness, which are influenced by happy hormones. Fertility is the concept of a happy reproductive system—encompassing libido, attraction, moods and ability to love. This is the foundation of life-long happiness for all couples.

If you've followed the guidelines set out in this book, you'll also see your weight come back in check. You'll be on the fast track to feeling amazing.

If for any reason you're struggling to get the basics down, or if it seems a bit too hard or confusing, there are plenty of trained health practitioners out there to help you take your wellness in hand.

I'm so pleased to have been given this chance to help you on your journey to wellness, to get fertile, grow babies and be well.

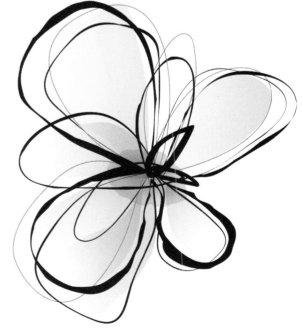

BIBLIOGRAPHY

Better Health Channel, 'Polycystic Ovarian Syndrome', February 2014, www. betterhealth.vic.gov.au/bhcv2/bhcarticles.nsf/pages/Polycystic_ovarian_ syndrome (viewed February 2014).

Eden, John, *Polycystic Ovary Syndrome: A Woman's Guide to Identifying and Managing PCOS,* Allen & Unwin, Sydney, 2005.

Kringoudis, Nat, 'Control Your Genes and Bubble Wrap Yourself from Cancer: My Interview with the Bruce Lipton', June 2014, www.natkringoudis.com. au/2013/06/control-your-genes-and-bubble-wrap-yourself-from-cancer-my- interview-with-the-bruce-lipton/ (viewed June 2014).

Lyttleton, Jane, *Treatment of Infertility with Chinese Medicine*, Churchill Livingstone, London, 2004.

Pope, Alexandra and Jane Bennett, *The Pill: Are You Sure It's for You?*, Allen & Unwin, Sydney, 2008.

Sadeghi, Habib, TED talk, 2 January 2014, www.youtube.com/ watch?v=y6yDk9Hky9o (viewed February 2014).

ACKNOWLEDGEMENTS

The process of writing this book has been one amazing journey. What started out as a very small e-book half the size of *Well & Good* very quickly grew up. I'm so proud of her.

I knew with every part of my body that this message needed to filter out there and that it was up to me to create a wave of change and shift the mindset of how we are currently approaching women's health. Now we've created the cherry on top—that this beautiful book will appeal to all women, young and old.

Thank you to the beautifully supportive team at my clinic, The Pagoda Tree. I rely on these inspiring souls to beat the drum of my message daily.

Thank you to my amazing team of personal staff—Amy, Rebecca and Sarah—and my manager and friend Sarah. It takes a strong bunch of like-minded people to make all that I do happen. You are collectively like rare precious stones and I'm never letting you go! (Okay, you can go for a short while to have your babies.)

Thank you to my life-changing business coach Lara. You have stretched me inside out and back to front and I'm forever grateful for you and all that you do.

Special thanks to Chamilka—you always make me look good and it's so appreciated.

Thanks to my production manager and very first editor, Ian. *Well & Good* is what it is because you believed we could make it so darn good even an 'old man' (your words!) could understand it. I'll never forget the day you said to me, if you can help me understand this 'stuff' you can help anybody. Seems we did it!

To my wellness sistas—you are a constant inspiration, and there are just so many of you. Jess, Mel and Sam—you all need a mention. We've supported each other in such amazing ways. Thank you.

Thank you to MUP for the opportunity to allow me to be creative, picky, fussy and pedantic. You too are a special bunch and I now know why we came together. I was told time and time again that publishing a book wasn't a pleasant experience. You've proven them all wrong—it's been an absolute delight.

And the biggest thank you to my family: To my ever-supportive husband Chris and incredible children Olivia and Geordie—you are my reason. To my parents Carol and Carl for giving me an upbringing for which I'm forever grateful and that paved the way to alternative health care. You both engrained in me that I could do anything. Always. To my sister Hollie and her family for being my number-one supporters and for constantly reminding me of the kind of person I want to be— you are true beauties.

And finally to all who will read this book. To the mothers I may inspire to pass this onto their daughters, the sisters who see the upmost value in sharing and the friends who love their pals so much they want to make everybody's day brighter and lighter. To the followers who have too come on this journey, I am forever grateful.

I pledge to continue to be the change I wish to see in this world and feel encouraged by the bountiful opportunities that lie ahead.

INDEX

RECIPE INDEX

MELBOURNE UNIVERSITY PRESS
An imprint of Melbourne University Publishing Limited
11–15 Argyle Place South, Carlton, Victoria 3053, Australia
mup-info@unimelb.edu.au
www.mup.com.au

First published 2014
Text © Natalie Kringoudis, 2014
Design and typography © Melbourne University Publishing Limited, 2014

Designed and typeset by Jacqueline Richards, PinchMe Design
Printed in China by 1010 Printing International Ltd

National Library of Australia Cataloguing-in-Publication entry

Kringoudis, Natalie, author.
Well & good: a woman's guide to a bountiful body/Nat Kringoudis.

9780522866766 (paperback)

Includes index.

Women—Health and hygiene
Self-care, Health.
Health behavior.
Nutrition.
Diet.
Exercise.

613.0424